Case Histories
Data Interpretations
for MRCP Examinations

Case Histories and Data Interpretations for MRCP Examinations

Christopher Chan
MB BCh, MD (Wales), FRCP (Glasgow), FRCP (London)
Consultant Physician
Basildon University Hospital
Nethermayne
Basildon, United Kingdom

Udayaraj Umasankar
MB BS, DTRD, MRCP (UK)
Staff Physician
Basildon University Hospital
Nethermayne
Basildon, United Kingdom

Farhad Huwez
MB ChB, PhD (Glasgow), MRCPI, FRCP (Glasgow)
Consultant Physician
Basildon University Hospital
Nethermayne
Basildon, United Kingdom

JAYPEE BROTHERS
MEDICAL PUBLISHERS (P) LTD
New Delhi

Published by
Jitendar P Vij
Jaypee Brothers Medical Publishers (P) Ltd
EMCA House, 23/23B Ansari Road, Daryaganj
New Delhi 110 002, India
Phones: 23272143, 23272703, 23282021, 23245672, 23245683
Fax: 011-23276490   e-mail: jpmedpub@del2.vsnl.net.in
Visit our website: http://www.jpbros.20m.com

Branches

• 202 Batavia Chambers, 8 Kumara Kruppa Road, Kumara Park East
  Bangalore 560 001, Phones: 2285971, 2382956 Tele Fax: 2281761
  e-mail: jaypeebc@bgl.vsnl.net.in

• 282 IIIrd Floor, Khaleel Shirazi Estate, Fountain Plaza
  Pantheon Road, **Chennai** 600 008, Phone: 28262665 Fax: 28262331
  e-mail: jpmedpub@md3.vsnl.net.in

• 4-2-1067/1-3, Ist Floor, Balaji Building, Ramkote Cross Road
  Hyderabad 500 095, Phones: 55610020, 24758498   Fax: 24758499
  e-mail: jpmedpub@rediffmail.com

• 1A Indian Mirror Street, Wellington Square
  Kolkata 700 013, Phone: 22451926 Fax: 22456075
  e-mail: jpbcal@cal.vsnl.net.in

• 106 Amit Industrial Estate, 61 Dr SS Rao Road, Near MGM Hospital
  Parel, **Mumbai** 400 012, Phones: 24124863, 24104532 Fax: 24160828
  e-mail: jpmedpub@bom7.vsnl.net.in

Case Histories and Data Interpretations for MRCP Examinations

First Edition: **2003**

Publishing Director: RK Yadav

ISBN 81-8061-158-2

Typeset at   JPBMP typesetting unit
Printed at   Gopsons Papers Ltd., Sector 60, Noida

Dedication

to
Our Families

Preface

'Real knowledge is to know the extent of one's ignorance.'
Confucius 551-479 BC

This book is intended to help doctors pass postgraduate examinations. The emphasis is on problem solving. We have deliberately included a number of difficult clinical cases and several new medical syndromes, which are not adequately described in standard medical textbooks. To tax our readers further we have included data interpretation generated by the panoply of diagnostic tests that are available in any modern hospital. The answers in this book reflect this eclectic mix of clinical cases and contain elaborate descriptions of new syndromes and concise details for less esoteric material. Clinical medicine is constantly evolving and changing and, therefore, for any future edition we would warmly welcome constructive comments on any of our clinical cases.

Christopher Chan
Udayaraj Umasankar
Farhad Huwez

Contents

Contents

Abbreviations

A&E	Accident and Emergency
ACE-I	Angiotensin Converting Enzyme Inhibitor
ACTH	Adrenocorticotrophic Hormone
ADH	Antidiuretic Hormone
AF	Atrial Fibrillation
ALP	Alkaline Phosphatase
ALT	Alanine Aminotransferase
ANA	Antinuclear Antibody
ANCA	Antineutrophilic Cytoplasmic Antibody
APTT	Activated Partial Thromboplastin Time
ARDS	Adult Respiratory Distress Syndrome
AST	Aspartate Aminotransferase
bd	*bis die* (twice daily)
BMI	Body Mass Index
BP	Blood Pressure
bpm	beats per minute
CCU	Coronary Care Unit
CHD	Coronary Heart Disease
CK	Creatine Kinase
COPD	Chronic Obstructive Pulmonary Disease
CRP	C-Reactive Protein
CSF	Cerebrospinal Fluid
CSU	Catheter specimen of urine
CT	Computed Tomography
CXR	Chest X-ray
DLCO	Diffusion Capacity of Lung for Carbon Monoxide
DNA	Deoxyribonucleic acid
DVT	Deep venous thrombosis
ECG	Electrocardiogram
ECHO	Echocardiogram
EEG	Electroencephalogram
e.g.	*exempli gratia* (for example)
ENT	Ear, Nose & Throat Department
EPO	Erythropoietin
ERCP	Endoscopic Retrograde Cholangiopancreatography
ESR	Erythrocyte Sedimentation Rate
FEV1	Forced Expiratory Volume in one second
FEV%	Forced Expiratory Volume as per cent of Vital Capacity
FSH	Follicle Stimulating Hormone
FBC	Full Blood Count

FVC	Forced Vital Capacity
γ-GT	Gamma-Glutamyl Transpeptidase
GH	Growth Hormone
GTN	Glyceryl Trinitrate
Hb	Haemoglobin
HbA_{1c}	Glycated Haemoglobin
HCO_3	Bicarbonate
HDL	High Density Lipoprotein
HIV	Human Immunodeficiency Virus
IgG	Immunoglobulin G
IGF	Insulin Like Growth Factor
IgM	Immunoglobulin M
INR	International Normalised Ratio
ITU	Intensive Therapy Unit
IV	Intravenous
IVC	Inferior Vena Cava
KCO	Diffusion Constant (DLCO/VA)
KHz	Kilohertz
LDL	Low Density Lipoprotein
LFT	Liver Function Tests
LH	Luteinising Hormone
LVF	Left Ventricular Failure
MCH	Mean Corpuscular Haemoglobin
MCHC	Mean Corpuscular Haemoglobin Concentration
MCV	Mean Corpuscular Volume
MI	Myocardial infarction
mmHg	millimetre of mercury
MRA	Magnetic Resonance Angiography
MRI	Magnetic Resonance Imaging
MSU	Mid Stream Urine
N.B.	*nota bene* (note well, or take notice)
NSAID	Non-steroidal Anti-inflammatory Drug
od	*omni die* (daily)
OGTT	Oral glucose tolerance test
$PaCO_2$	Arterial Carbon Dioxide
PaO_2	Arterial Oxygen
PEFR	Peak Expiratory Flow Rate
PO_4	Serum Phosphate
PSA	Prostate Specific Antigen
PTH	Parathyroid Hormone
RBBB	Right Bundle Branch Block
ref	Reference value (s)
RV	Residual Lung Volume
SIADH	Syndrome of Inappropriate ADH secretion
s/c	Subcutaneous
SLE	Systemic Lupus Erythematosus

SVC	Static Vital Capacity
TB	Tuberculosis
TBG	Thyroid Binding Globulin
tds	*ter die sumendus* (three times daily)
TIA	Transient ischaemic attack
TNF	Tumour Necrosis Factor
TRH	Thyrotropin Releasing Hormone
TSH	Thyroid Stimulating Hormone
TLC	Total Lung Capacity
tPA	Tissue Plasminogen Activator
U & E	Urea and Electrolytes
VA	Alveolar Volume
VC	Vital capacity
VLDL	Very Low Density Lipoprotein
WBC	White Blood Cell count

Recommended International Non-proprietary Name (rINN)

The European directive 92/27/EEC requires the use of Recommended International Non-proprietary Name (rINN) for medicinal substances. In most instances the British Approved Name (BAN) and the Recommended International Non-proprietary Name (rINN) differ slightly in spelling. A complete list of substances with proposed name changes is available from the British National Formulary website: www.bnf.org.uk. The following table gives the British Approved Name (BAN) and the Recommended International Non-proprietary Name (rINN) for some of the drugs quoted in this book. For the correct doses of all drugs and their approved name, please consult your local formulary.

BAN	rINN
adrenaline	epinephrine
amoxycillin	amoxicillin
amphetamine	amfetamine
bendrofluazide	bendroflumethiazide
busulphan	busulfan
cholestyramine	colestyramine
corticotrophin	corticotropin
cyclosporin	ciclosporin
dothiepin	dosulepin
frusemide	furosemide
hydroxyurea	hydroxycarbamide
noradrenaline	norepinephrine
oestradiol	estradiol
oxpentifylline	pentoxifylline
phenobarbitone	phenobarbital
thyroxine	levothyroxine
sulphasalazine	sulfasalazine

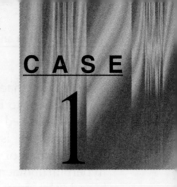

CASE 1

CASE 1

A 66-year-old man was admitted with a left cerebral infarct. The initial blood tests were:

Hb	11.5 g/dl
WBC	$5.0 \times 10^9/l$
Platelets	$167 \times 10^9/l$
Bilirubin	16 μmol/l
ALT	16 U/l
ALP	32 U/l
CRP	< 8 mg/l

Two weeks later he developed jaundice. At this stage the repeat blood tests were as follows:

Hb	7.1 g/dl
WBC	$6.2 \times 10^9/l$
Platelets	$369 \times 10^9/l$
Bilirubin	38 μmol/l
MCV	86.1 fl
MCH	30.5 pg
MCHC	35.4 g/dl
Na	139 mmol/l
K	3.5 mmol/l
Urea	9.0 mmol/l
Creatinine	91 μmol/l
Glucose	5.7 mmol/l
CRP	107 mg/l
ALT	116 U/l
ALP	12 U/l
Blood film	polychromasia, anisocytosis and spherocytosis
Coagulation screen	normal
Direct antiglobulin test	negative
Ultrasound abdomen	14.5 cm enlarged spleen

Question

What type of anaemia is this? Give two likely causes?

Answer

Non-immune haemolytic anaemia:
* secondary to infection
* drug induced

Haemolysis is the destruction of red cells, which can be intravascular or extravascular. It results in unconjugated hyperbilirubinaemia and secondary reticulocytosis. Hence, the blood film may show macrocytosis and polychromasia. Spherocytosis occurs in certain types of haemolytic anaemias. Intravascular haemolysis leads to reduced plasma haptoglobin and haemopoxin levels, but elevated lactate dehydrogenase. The plasma contains increased levels of methaemoglobin and free haemoglobin. Breakdown products of haemoglobin appear in the urine as haemoglobinuria and haemosiderinuria.

Haemolytic anaemias can be inherited or acquired. Inherited causes include red cell membrane defects (hereditary spherocytosis), red cell metabolic disorders (G6PD deficiency) and haemoglobinopathies (thalassaemias, sickle cell anaemias).

Acquired haemolytic anaemias can be of immune or non-immune origin. In immune haemolytic anaemias antibodies are formed against red cells and hence the direct antiglobulin (Coombs') test is positive. Antibodies are classified into warm and cold type depending on the temperature at which they are most active against the red cells. Warm antibodies are most active at body temperature and these occur in the following conditions:

a. Primary. Evan's syndrome describes the combination of haemolysis and thrombocytopenia.

b. Secondary such as in SLE, chronic lymphatic leukaemia, lymphomas.

Cold agglutinins are found in idiopathic cold haemagglutinin disease, lymphomas particularly histiocytic types, paroxysmal cold haemoglobinuria, infectious mononucleosis, mycoplasmal infections and some viral infections.

Drugs such as such as methyldopa and levodopa can cause autoimmune haemolysis. This usually requires a long exposure to the drug (3-6 months) and the anaemia is extravascular. Drugs such as isoniazid and rifampicin form immune complexes and the anaemia is intravascular.

Non-immune haemolytic anaemias are seen in conditions like microangiopathic haemolytic anaemia (MAHA), paroxysmal nocturnal haemoglobinuria (PNH), and mechanical damage (e.g. from prosthetic heart valves).

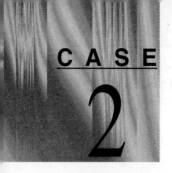

CASE 2

A 45-year-old lady presented with tingling sensation and cramps in her hands. Initial screening showed the following results:

Corrected calcium	1.37 mmol/l
PO_4	1.59 mmol/l
Albumin	48 g/l
ALP	69 U/l
Na	135 mmol/l
K	4.0 mmol/l
Urea	7.0 mmol/l
Creatinine	121 μmol/l

Questions

1. What is the most likely cause of her hypocalcaemia?
2. Name two clinical signs associated with hypocalcaemia?
3. What is the ECG finding associated with hypocalcaemia?

Answers

1. Idiopathic hypoparathyroidism
2. Chvostek's sign and Trousseau's sign
3. Prolonged QT interval

Hypocalcaemia produces neuromuscular irritability, which presents with tingling sensation, tetany, mental changes, convulsions, and laryngeal stridor. One should also look for Chvostek's sign (facial twitching produced by tapping the facial nerve) and Trousseau's sign (muscular spasm of the fingers induced by a sphygmomanometer cuff applied on the upper arm and held above diastolic blood pressure for 3 minutes). Cataracts occur with chronic hypocalcaemia.

Causes of Hypocalcaemia

- Renal disease
- Hypoparathyroidism
- Pseudohypoparathyroidism
- Vitamin D deficiency
- Drugs (Bisphosphonates)
- Acute pancreatitis

Investigations in hypocalcaemia should include:
- Renal function
- Serum chloride, bicarbonate and phosphate levels
- Parathyroid hormone levels
- Vitamin D levels

N.B. A low calcium and high phosphate can occur with:
- Hypoparathyroidism
- Renal disease

The treatment of hypocalcaemia consists of replacing calcium by the oral or parenteral route and administering vitamin D.

Hypoparathyroidism

The diagnosis of hypoparathyroidism is based on low serum calcium and high phosphate with normal renal function and the absence of osteomalacia or malabsorption. The causes of hypoparathyroidism are:
- Familial (autosomal dominant or recessive)
- Autoimmune

Hypoparathyroidism co-existing with Addison's disease is part of the Type 1 polyglandular syndrome.

- Surgical (thyroidectomy, parathyroidectomy)
- Hypomagnesaemia (low magnesium interferes with PTH secretion)
- DiGeorge's syndrome (congenital absence of parathyroid tissue)

Pseudohypoparathyroidism

Pseudohypoparathyroidism is due to end organ resistance to PTH. There are two types of pseudohypoparathyroidism:

- Type 1A is an autosomal dominant condition associated with intellectual failure and Albright's osteodystrophy (short stature, round face, short neck, short digits [brachydactyly], and subcutaneous calcifications). In this form of pseudohypoparathyroidism, the failure of tissues to respond to PTH is due to loss of G protein, which couples the PTH receptor to adenyl cyclase. This G protein couples many other hormone receptors to adenyl cyclase and thus account for resistance to TSH, LH and FSH.

  Pseudo-pseudo-hypoparathyroidism refers to the presence of Albright's osteodystrophy and loss of G protein, but without hypocalcaemia.

- Type 1B is an isolated resistance to PTH, G protein is normal, and mechanism is as yet unknown. The inheritance is also unclear.

CASE 3

A 48-year-old man presented with acute weakness of the right arm and leg. No other focal neurological deficit was identified. His pulse was regular at 72 bpm and BP 128/68 mmHg. He did not smoke cigarettes or drink alcohol. Two years ago he was treated for a deep vein thrombosis of the left leg with heparin for one week and subsequently took warfarin for three months. His full blood count, serum electrolytes, and coagulation studies were normal. The ESR was 13 mm/h, glucose 4.9 mmol/l, and cholesterol 5.4 mmol/l. The ECG confirmed sinus rhythm and there were no arrhythmias on 24 hour ECG monitoring. A transthoracic echocardiogram showed no intra-cardiac thrombi or valvular heart disease. Chest X-ray was unremarkable. A CT brain showed a low attenuation area in the frontoparietal region of the left cerebral hemisphere. Doppler ultrasound did not reveal any stenosis in the carotid or vertebral arteries. The Protein C, Protein S (free) and Antithrombin III levels were normal. The serology for vasculitis and rheumatoid disease were negative. Lupus anticoagulant was not demonstrated. The anticardiolipin IgG antibody was raised at 82 GPLU/ml (ref 0-20), but the anticardiolipin IgM antibody was not detected.

Questions
1. What is the most likely cause of this ischaemic stroke?
2. How is this condition is treated?

Answers
1. Primary antiphospholipid syndrome
2. Oral anticoagulation

Antiphospholipid Syndrome

The antiphospholipid antibodies comprise a heterogeneous family of antibodies directed against phospholipids, including anticardiolipin antibody (aCL) and lupus anticoagulant (LA). They are associated with a hypercoagulable state and manifestations include thrombosis, foetal loss, thrombocytopenia, sterile endocarditis with embolism, and a variety of neurological conditions. These antibodies are either IgG or IgM and the former (IgG) is frequently associated with thrombosis. Antiphospholipid syndrome (APS) may be diagnosed when arterial or venous thrombosis, or recurrent miscarriage occurs in a subject in whom laboratory tests for antiphospholipid antibodies (aCL, LA or both) are positive. The commonest neurological conditions associated with APS include amaurosis fugax, multiple cerebral infarctions, dementia, transient ischaemic attacks (TIAs), and Guillain-Barré syndrome. Patients with cerebral infarcts associated with APS tend to be young individuals with a slight preponderance of females. The most common site of thrombosis is in the deep veins of the leg. Cerebral thrombosis is the most frequent arterial lesion and 20% of all thrombosis tends to involve the cerebral circulation. However, cerebral infarction can be a consequence of arterial or venous occlusion. A high recurrence rate for stroke and TIA was also shown in patients with cerebral ischaemia and positive antiphospholipid antibodies.

The guidelines of the British Society of Haematology's Haemostasis and Thrombosis Task Force recommend the testing of young patients with strokes for antiphospholipid antibodies. This can be extended to older people who present with strokes in the absence of cardiovascular risk factors. Thromboembolic disease and miscarriage are common in the general population and antiphospholipid antibodies can be transient. For these reasons, the persistence of positive antiphospholipid results must be demonstrated in separate samples collected at least six weeks apart. A careful search for connective tissue disorders is needed to exclude secondary antiphospholipid syndrome. For cerebral infarction in the antiphospholipid syndrome these guidelines recommend long term oral anticoagulant therapy with an optimal INR range of 2.0-3.0 due to the high recurrence rate.

Secondary Causes of Antiphospholipid Syndrome

- Rheumatoid arthritis
- Systemic sclerosis
- Systemic lupus erythematosus
- Temporal arteritis
- Sjögren's syndrome
- Behçet's syndrome
- Psoriatic arthropathy

Other Causes of Positive Antiphospholipid Antibodies

- Viral i.e. HIV, varicella, hepatitis C
- Bacterial such as syphilis
- Parasitic i.e. malaria
- Malignant lymphoma, paraproteinaemia, autoimmune thrombocytopenia and autoimmune haemolytic anaemia.
- Drug exposure such as phenothiazines, procainamide, phenytoin, quinidine and hydralazine.
- Intravenous drug abuse
- Livedo reticularis
- Guillain-Barré syndrome

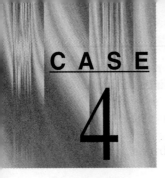

CASE

4

CASE 4

A 47-year-old solicitor presented to his General Practitioner with a 2 months history of back pain that radiated into both thighs. There was no history of trauma. He admitted to dribbling micturition and erectile dysfunction for the past two weeks. Past medical history included peptic ulcer disease. He was on co-dydramol and cimetidine. On examination, there was mild weakness of the legs (power 4/5), exaggerated knee and ankle jerks in both legs, and a right extensor plantar response. After 2 days in hospital, he developed urinary retention and a left sided lower motor neurone facial palsy. Chest X-ray showed consolidation in the right upper zone.

ESR	72 mm/h
Hb	12.3 g/dl
WBC	11.9 x 10⁹/l
Platelets	411 x 10⁹/l
Na	132 mmol/l
K	4.8 mmol/l
Urea	4.3 mmol/l
Creatinine	92 µmol/l
Glucose	6.4 mmol/l
Bilirubin	18 µmol/l
AST	21 U/l
ALT	20 U/l
ALP	430 U/l
Albumin	36 g/l
Urinalysis	normal

Arterial Blood Gases (on air)

pH	7.4
PaCO$_2$	4.3 kPa
PaO$_2$	8.5 kPa
HCO$_3$	30 mmol/l

Blood cultures grew Staphylococcus aureus. He was commenced on oxygen and IV antibiotics.

Questions
1. List 4 conditions that have to be excluded.
2. What initial measures are essential for his management?
3. What other tests are needed to reach the final diagnosis?

Answers

1. The following conditions need to be excluded:
   - Guillain-Barré syndrome
   - Acute intermittent porphyria
   - Vasculitis
   - Sarcoidosis

2. The following initial measures are necessary for his management:
   - Admit the patient to ITU
   - Measurements of PEFR and FEV1
   - Urinary porphyrins
   - Lumbar puncture and CSF examination

3. This patient has an ascending paralysis and evidence of a multisystem disease with pulmonary and hepatic involvement. For this reason a collagen vascular disease and sarcoidosis need to be excluded. The essential diagnostic tests are:
   - Autoantibody screen (ANA, DNA binding test and ANCA).
   - Repeat chest X-ray after antibiotic therapy, followed if appropriate by CT chest.
   - Bronchoscopy and bronchial lavage for TB, atypical infections, cytology. Bronchoscopic or transbronchial biopsy has superseded the Kveim test.
   - Kveim test. This test material is taken from the spleen of a patient with sarcoidosis. It is injected intradermally and the skin site is biopsied 4-6 weeks later. A positive test is the appearance of typical sarcoid granulomas. In the UK there are concerns over the theoretical risks of transmitting Creutzfeldt-Jakob disease by the Kveim test material, which has now been withdrawn by the manufacturers. Elsewhere in the world the Kveim test is restricted to patients in whom it is not possible to obtain diagnostic tissue samples, e.g. neurosarcoidosis.
   - Angiotensin-converting enzyme (ACE) in the serum or CSF. ACE is produced by sarcoid granulomas and elevated serum levels are seen in 60% of sarcoid patients, but these do not correlate with disease activity or response to treatment. Serum ACE levels have poor diagnostic sensitivity (60%) and specificity (60%), because elevated levels occur in many disorders, including TB, leprosy, primary biliary cirrhosis, and diabetes.
   - Mantoux test
   - MRI scan of the spine to exclude a focal lesion

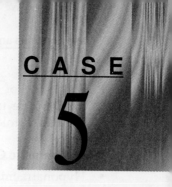

CASE
5

CASE 5

A 78-year-old lady presented with dyspnoea and lethargy. She has never smoked cigarettes. Chest X-ray showed a prominent left hilum.

Na	115 mmol/l
K	4.8 mmol/l
Urea	3.0 mmol/l
Creatinine	80 μmol/l
Glucose	6.0 mmol/l
Plasma osmolality	240 mosmol/kg
Urine osmolality	625 mosmol/kg
Urine Na	35 mmol/l

The full blood count, thyroid function test, calcium and cholesterol levels were normal. A short Synacthen test showed a normal response. Gonadotrophin levels were elevated and in keeping with her postmenopausal state. CT chest showed a 5 cm irregular mass in the left hilum that had extended into the adjacent lung tissues.

Questions

1. Why is there a low serum sodium?
2. What is the complete diagnosis?
3. What other investigations would you undertake?

Answers

1. Syndrome of Inappropriate ADH secretion (SIADH)
2. SIADH due to left bronchogenic carcinoma
3. Sputum cytology, bronchoscopy

The Diagnostic Criteria for SIADH

- Hyponatraemia with plasma hypo-osmolality (< 270 mosmol/kg).
- High urine osmolality (i.e. higher than plasma).
- Continued renal sodium excretion (urine Na > 30 mmol/1).
- Absence of hypotension, hypovolaemia, and oedematous states (heart failure, cirrhosis, nephrotic syndrome).
- Normal renal, adrenal and thyroid function.

The Causes of SIADH

- Pulmonary (small cell lung tumour, lung abscess, pneumonia, TB)
- Drugs (carbamazepine, cyclophosphamide, thiazides, Ecstasy)
- CNS (head injury, subdural haematoma, meningitis, subarachnoid haemorrhage)
- Metabolic (porphyria, alcohol withdrawal, post operative)
  Treatment of SIADH is by either fluid restriction or demeclocycline, or in acute symptomatic cases, i.e. patients presenting with coma and convulsions, by hypertonic (3%) saline. However, too rapid correction of hyponatraemia may precipitate central pontine myelinolysis.
- In asymptomatic patients with chronic hyponatraemia, the correction rate should not be faster than 0.5 mmol/1 per hour and not more than 10 mmol/1 per 24 hours.
- In acute symptomatic hyponatraemia, the correction rate should not be faster than 2 mmol/1 per hour and not more than 25 mmol/1 in the first 24 hours.

Hypertonic (3% saline)

The use of hypertonic (3%) saline is reserved for hyponatraemic patients with coma or convulsions. This treatment should be used with the utmost care. Sodium levels must be measured 2 hourly. To arrest seizure activity, it is only necessary to raise the serum sodium level by 4-6 mmol/l. The calculation for the rate of sodium replacement is illustrated below:

- 3% hypertonic saline = 513 mmol of sodium per litre. (compared with 0.9% saline = 150 mmol of sodium per litre).

- Rate of sodium replacement (mmol per hour) = Total Body Water × desired correction rate (mmol/l per hour).

- Total Body Water = 60% of body weight in kg
  E.g. 70 kg adult and a correction rate of 0.5 mmol/l per hour:
  Rate of sodium replacement
  = 60% × 70 kg × 0.5 mmol/l per hour
  = 21 mmol per hour
  = 21 × $\frac{1000}{513}$ = 41 ml per hour of 3% saline

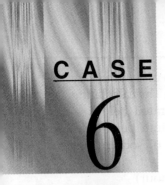

C A S E

6

CASE 6

An 80-year-old lady was referred to the haematology clinic. Clinically she was pale, the chest was clear, and there was no hepatosplenomegaly. A systolic murmur was heard over the aortic area.

Hb	7.5 g/dl
WBC	$9.0 \times 10^9/l$
Platelets	$250 \times 10^9/l$
MCV	93.8 fl
MCH	30.2 pg

The blood film showed burr cells, schistocytes and spherocytes. Liver function tests and serum protein electrophoresis were normal. The bone marrow showed dyserythropoiesis, iron stores were present, and more than 15% of erythroblasts were ring sideroblasts.

Questions
1. What is the cause of her anaemia?
2. How would you treat this patient?

Answers
1. Myelodysplasia (refractory anaemia with ringed sideroblasts).
2. Transfusion.

Myelodysplasia or myelodysplastic syndrome (MDS) refers to a heterogeneous group of bone marrow disorders characterised by ineffective erythropoiesis, peripheral blood cytopenias and a tendency for leukaemic transformation. It is common among the elderly; the incidence is 22 per 100,000 in those over the age of 70 years. MDS is one cause of an unexplained macrocytosis in elderly patients.

Aetiology of MDS
- Chromosomal abnormalities are common, e.g. deletions in the long arm of chromosome 5 (5q-) which contain important genes for granulocyte-macrophage colony-stimulating factor (GM-CSF) and other growth factors.
- MDS can occur in cancer patients who had received chemotherapy or radiotherapy many years previously. This type of MDS progresses rapidly to leukaemia.

FAB (French-American-British) Classification
In the FAB classification MDS is grouped into:
- Refractory anaemia (RA)
- Refractory anaemia with ringed sideroblasts (RARS)
- Refractory anaemia with excess blast cells (RAEB)
- Refractory anaemia with excess blast cells in transformation (RAEB-t)
- Chronic myelomonocytic leukaemia (CML)

The diagnosis is based on the peripheral blood film and bone marrow findings:

	Bone Marrow Blasts %	Bone Marrow Ring sideroblasts %	Peripheral Blood Blasts %	Peripheral Blood Monocytes %
RA	≤ 5	< 15	≤ 1	-
RARS	≤ 5	> 15	≤ 1	-
CML	≤ 20	-	< 5	$> 1 \times 10^9/l$
RAEB	5-20	-	< 5	-
RAEB-t	>20-30 ± Auer rods	-	> 5	-

Bournemouth Score

The Bournemouth score provides prognostic information and is based on the following features, each of which is given a score of 1:

- Bone marrow blasts $\geq 5\%$
- Haemoglobin ≤ 10 g/dl
- Neutrophils $\leq 2.5 \times 10^9/l$
- Platelets $\leq 100 \times 10^9/l$

From the total score, the median survival can be predicted.

Bournemouth Score	Grade	Predicted median survival
0-1	A	62 months
2-3	B	22 months
4	C	8.5 months

Cytogenetic features are now regarded as important for prognostic prediction and are incorporated in the International Prognosis Scoring System (IPSS). In the IPSS good prognostic features are: normal karyotype, deletions in the long arm of chromosome 5 (5q-), and deletions in the long arm of chromosome 20 (20q-). Abnormalities in chromosome 7 and multiple chromosomal abnormalities have a poorer outlook.

Treatment of MDS

- Supportive measures for anaemia, infection, and bleeding.
- Chemotherapy is given in low doses to abolish abnormal blast cells and is followed by growth factors to stimulate marrow cell lines to differentiate.
- Allogeneic bone marrow transplantation.
- Growth factors. Granulocyte-macrophage colony-stimulating factor (GM-CSF), Granulocyte colony-stimulating factor (G-CSF), erythropoietin and thrombopoietin, which target myeloid, erythroid and megakaryoid precursors, respectively. Other agents that may induce cellular differentiation are interleukins, interferons, vitamin D3, and retinoic acid.

CASE 7

This is the audiogram of a 50-year-old man with impaired hearing.

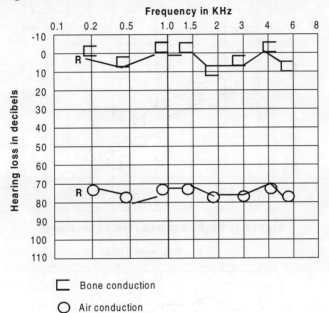

Frequency in KHz

⊏ Bone conduction

◯ Air conduction

Questions

1. What does the audiogram show?
2. What is the diagnosis?
3. Give two possible causes.

Answers

1. Impaired auditory acuity in the right ear for air conduction.
2. Conductive deafness right ear.
3. Chronic otitis media. Wax in the external ear.

Audiograms are a subjective way of assessing hearing. Different sound frequencies are delivered at varying intensity levels to assess air conduction (AC) and bone conduction (BC). The results are plotted in a graph where the sound

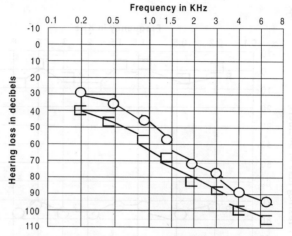

Figure 1: Right ear age related deafness

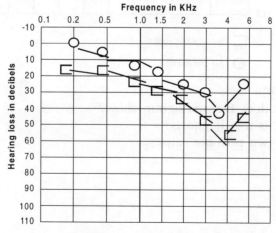

Figure 2: Right ear noise related deafness

frequency is shown along the X-axis and the **hearing loss in decibels** along the Y-axis. The following symbols are used:

	Right ear	Left ear
AC	O	X
BC	[	]

In healthy individuals AC is better than BC. In conductive deafness AC is impaired, but BC is intact and, therefore, the audiogram will show an air-bone gap (see Figure in the Question 7). In sensorineural deafness AC and BC are affected equally and, therefore, the audiogram will not show an air-bone gap (Figure 1, 2).

Conductive deafness is produced by external ear or middle ear pathology. Sensorineural deafness can be age related if it is bilateral, but suggests a cerebellopontine angle lesion such as a meningioma or acoustic neuroma if it is unilateral.

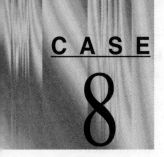

C A S E

8

CASE 8

A 75-year-old lady presented with lethargy and constipation. Her thyroid function tests showed the following:

TSH	9.43 mU/l
Free T4	7.8 pmol/l

The thyroid peroxidase antibody was positive in a titre of 1 in 245.

Question

1. What is the diagnosis?

Answer

The tests show a raised serum TSH in the presence of a low T4, which is consistent with the diagnosis of primary hypothyroidism. The presence of thyroid peroxidase (TPO) antibody in high titre indicates autoimmune thyroid disease, i.e. Hashimoto's thyroiditis.

Thyroid Autoantibodies

- TPO antibody used to be called thyroid microsomal antibody.
- High titres of the TPO antibody suggest autoimmune thyroid disease.
- TPO antibody occurs in both forms of autoimmune thyroid disease, Hashimoto's thyroiditis and Graves' disease.
- TPO antibody does not give information on the thyroid status i.e. hypothyroid or hyperthyroid.
- TPO antibody titres will decrease with time following thyroxine treatment for Hashimoto's thyroiditis and antithyroid therapy in Graves' disease.
- Other types of thyroid autoantibodies are thyroglobulin (Tg) antibody and TSH receptor antibody (TSH-R), which may be stimulating or blocking in action. TSH-R stimulating antibody occurs in Graves' disease and used to be called long acting thyroid stimulator (LATS). TSH-R stimulating antibody can cross the placenta to induce neonatal hyperthyroidism. Placental transfer of the TSH-R blocking antibody can produce congenital hypothyroidism.

Hypothyroidism

Hypothyroidism results from underactivity of the thyroid gland. This can be primary (disease of thyroid gland), or secondary (disease of the pituitary). A low T4 with raised TSH points to primary hypothyroidism, whereas a low T4 with a low TSH suggests secondary hypothyroidism.

Causes of Primary Hypothyroidism

- Thyroidectomy.
- Radioiodine (10% of patients develop hypothyroidism in the first year after radioiodine treatment and the subsequent risk is about 5% per annum).

- Autoimmune thyroid disease (Hashimoto's thyroiditis).
- "Idiopathic"
- Antithyroid drugs (e.g. carbimazole, lithium).
- Iodine deficiency.
- Iodine in *excessive quantities* (e.g. radiocontrast dye, amiodarone) interferes with the iodination of TBG, which is called the Wolff-Chaikoff effect, and reduces thyroid hormone output.
- Subacute thyroiditis is sometimes called De Quervain's thyroiditis and is probably viral in aetiology. The thyroid gland is painful and the ESR is very high, but thyroid autoantibodies are absent. Thyroid gland inflammation and destruction result in thyroid hormone release and transient hyperthyroidism, which may be followed by permanent hypothyroidism in 10% of patients.
- Postpartum thyroiditis affects about 10% of women. These patients usually have positive thyroid autoantibodies. Hyperthyroidism in the first 4 months is followed by either complete recovery (i.e. euthyroidism), or transient hypothyroidism that require temporary thyroxine replacement. Postpartum thyroiditis can reappear in subsequent pregnancies. Eventually permanent hypothyroidism develops in about one third of these women, who will require life long thyroxine therapy.
- Congenital, e.g. Pendred's syndrome (hypothyroidism, goitre, and sensorineural deafness) is due to a partial defect in iodide organification. This means iodine is not incorporated into thyroglobulin and cannot be trapped within the thyroid gland. In this syndrome, iodide is easily released from the thyroid gland in response to potassium perchlorate.

Causes of Secondary Hypothyroidism

- Hypopituitarism due to pituitary adenoma
- Pituitary surgery or radiotherapy

The most common form of primary hypothyroidism in adults is Hashimoto's thyroiditis, which is associated with other autoimmune diseases including Type 2 and Type 3 polyglandular syndromes. Primary "idiopathic" hypothyroidism refers to the thyroid gland failure associated with end stage autoimmune thyroid disease (Hashimoto's thyroiditis, or burnt out Graves' disease). The clinical features of hypothyroidism include lethargy, cold intolerance, bradycardia, constipation, and weight gain. Severe hypothyroidism in the elderly can present as myxoedema coma with hypothermia. These patients need to be managed in the ITU with gradual warming, oxygen, thyroxine replacement, intravenous hydrocortisone and monitoring for hypoglycaemia.

Rare forms of hypothyroidism are produced by hypothalamic TRH deficiency (so called tertiary hypothyroidism) and resistance of peripheral tissues to the action of thyroid hormone (Refetoff's syndrome). In the latter condition, T4 and T3 are elevated, TSH is normal or high, but the patient may be hypothyroid. This is due to a faulty thyroid hormone receptor, which is unable to bind effectively to T3.

Polyglandular Autoimmune Syndromes (PAS)

Autoimmune destruction of certain endocrine glands tends to occur together. The occurrence of one endocrine deficiency should, therefore, prompt a careful search for other components of a polyglandular syndrome. At present three categories of PAS are described.

Type 1 PAS

Type 1 PAS is also called Whitaker syndrome. It is an autosomal recessive condition with an abnormal gene on the short arm of chromosome 21. Type 1 PAS consists of at least two of the three following:
- Chronic mucocutaneous candidiasis
- Hypoparathyroidism
- Autoimmune adrenal insufficiency

These patients present before the age of 5 years with mucocutaneous candidiasis, followed by hypoparathyroidism before the age of 10 years and finally Addison's disease during the mid-teens. Other associated features are: Type 1 diabetes, hypogonadism, pernicious anaemia, and vitiligo.

Type 2 PAS

Type 2 PAS or Schmidt's syndrome consists of:

-25-

- Addison's disease with autoimmune thyroid disease (either Hashimoto's thyroiditis or Graves' disease).
- *Or*, Addison's disease with Type 1 diabetes

Type 2 PAS shows an autosomal dominant inheritance with incomplete penetrance and presents in the third or fourth decade of life. Other associated features are: hypopituitarism, primary hypogonadism, myasthenia gravis, Parkinson's disease, coeliac disease, pernicious anaemia, autoimmune thrombocytopenia, vitiligo.

Type 3 PAS

There are 3 varieties of Type 3 PAS:
- Type 3a. Autoimmune thyroiditis with Type 1 diabetes
- Type 3b. Autoimmune thyroiditis with pernicious anaemia
- Type 3c. Autoimmune thyroiditis with vitiligo, alopecia

Type 3 PAS is an autosomal dominant disorder with incomplete penetrance and occurs in middle age. Other associated features are: coeliac disease, hypogonadism, myasthenia gravis, sarcoidosis, rheumatoid disease, Sjögren's syndrome, gastric carcinoid, pancreatic steatorrhoea.

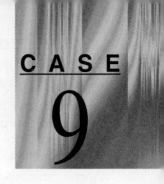
CASE 9

A 70-year-old lady was admitted to the CCU with syncope and angina. A cardiac murmur was found on examination. Cardiac catheterisation showed the following results:

Cardiac pressures

Left ventricle	195/15 mmHg
Aorta	121/72 mmHg

Coronary angiogram

60% stenosis of the obtuse marginal coronary artery and the mid portion of the right coronary artery.

Questions
1. What is the diagnosis?
2. What is the treatment?

Answers

1. Severe aortic stenosis and coronary artery disease.
2. Aortic valve replacement and coronary artery bypass graft (CABG) surgery.

Aortic Stenosis

Aortic stenosis presents with the following triad of symptoms: angina, breathlessness and syncope. The causes of aortic stenosis are:

Congenital

- Unicuspid valve. Symptoms occur during infancy and in children under 15 years.
- Bicuspid valve. Calcific stenosis often with regurgitation occurs after the fourth decade of life. A congenital bicuspid valve is the most common congenital cardiac abnormality and is seen in 0.4-2.0% of live births.

Acquired

- Senile degenerative calcification usually occurs in patients over the age of 65 years. Valvular stenosis is accelerated in diabetes mellitus and hypercholesterolaemia; co-existing coronary artery disease is common; calcification may also involve the mitral annulus and the conduction system leading to heart block.
- Rheumatic valve disease is now uncommon in developed countries.
- End-stage renal failure is associated with aortic stenosis, perhaps as a result of abnormal calcium and phosphate metabolism.
- Paget's disease, where the prevalence of aortic stenosis is four times higher than in the general population.
- Rheumatoid arthritis, SLE, radiation (rare causes)

Echocardiography of Aortic Stenosis

- The pressure gradient across the aortic valve is given by the modified Bernoulli's equation:
  Aortic valve gradient (mmHg) = $4 \times V^2$

V = velocity of the jet of blood across the stenotic valve, expressed as metres per second, is easily measured by Doppler.

The Doppler beam must be closely aligned to the flow across the valve; otherwise the gradient will be underestimated. The mean gradient is also underestimated in patients with a low cardiac output, and overestimated if the haemoglobin is less than 8 g/dl. Severe aortic stenosis is shown by a mean gradient of > 50 mmHg and an aortic valve area of < 1 cm^2 (normal aortic valve area is > 2.5 cm^2).

- The Aortic valve area (AVA) is given by the Continuity Equation:

  AVA = LVOT area x (LVOT-TVI ÷ AV-TVI)

  LVOT refers to left ventricular outflow tract.

  TVI indicates time velocity integral.

  Cardiac catheterisation may be necessary if there is doubt about the accuracy of the echocardiography data, and if there is concomitant coronary artery disease requiring bypass surgery. During cardiac catheterisation, the Gorlin equation allows the aortic valve area to be calculated from:

  AVA = LVOT area x (LVOT velocity ÷ aortic valve blood flow velocity)

- Other echocardiographic findings in aortic stenosis are

  Left ventricular hypertrophy

  Valve anatomy (tricuspid or bicuspid, and presence of calcification)

Treatment of Aortic Stenosis

- Aortic valve replacement, often with coronary artery bypass surgery.
- Aortic balloon valvuloplasty. This is used in young patients with stenosis of a non-calcified congenital bicuspid valve. It is of limited value in adults with calcific aortic stenosis and is contraindicated in patients who have concomitant aortic regurgitation. It is sometimes used as a palliative procedure for patients who are unfit for valve surgery and pregnant women, or is undertaken to stabilise critically ill patients before embarking on valve surgery. Complications include aortic regurgitation, aortic

perforation, stroke, and myocardial infarction. Restenosis is common in patients with severely dysplastic valves.

- Heart failure measures in those patients where surgery is not an option.
- Remember bacterial endocarditis prophylaxis.

Indications for Aortic Valve Replacement

- Severely symptomatic aortic stenosis
- Aortic stenosis with requiring CABG coronary artery disease
- Aortic stenosis with syncope on effort
- Surgery should also be considered if there is hypotension on exercise or diminished LV function.
- Other possible indications are: aortic stenosis with ventricular tachycardia, LVH, and aortic valve area < 0.6 cm^2.
- Bioprosthetic valves, unlike mechanical ones, do not require long term anticoagulation and are, therefore, preferred in the elderly.

Heyde's Syndrome

In 1958 Heyde first described bleeding from angiodysplasias of the colon among a group of 10 patients with calcific aortic stenosis. As both conditions are relatively common, their occurrence together in the same patient is arguably due to chance. Others have suggested an acquired von Willebrand's disease may be the cause of the bleeding diathesis. Aortic valve replacement may normalise the plasma von Willebrand levels and stop the bleeding tendency.

CASE 10

A 55-year-old man was admitted with a right hemiplegia and the CT brain scan confirmed a frontoparietal infarction of the left cerebral hemisphere. Three weeks later he collapsed while walking to toilet. His pulse was regular at 110 bpm and BP 96/64 mmHg. The heart sounds, chest, and abdomen were unremarkable on examination. There was no leg oedema. No new neurological signs were discovered. The ECG showed sinus rhythm. The chest X-ray did not show any abnormalities. Arterial blood gases and echocardiogram were done urgently.

Arterial blood gases (on air):

pH	7.4
PaO$_2$	8.64 kPa
PaCO$_2$	5.5 kPa
HCO$_3$	24.6 mmol/l
Base excess	- 2.4 mmol/l
Oxygen saturation	89%

Transthoracic echocardiogram
Severely dilated right heart with reduced systolic function. Severe tricuspid regurgitation.
Left ventricle showed good systolic function with reversed septal motion.
Normal left atrium.

Questions
1. What do the arterial blood gases show?
2. Why did he collapse?
3. What other investigation is required?

Answers

1. Type 1 respiratory failure
2. Pulmonary embolism
3. Radioisotope ventilation perfusion lung scan, or spiral CT chest.

CASE 11

A 40-year-old man was admitted to the ITU with drowsiness and hypotension. The heart rate was regular at 126 bpm, blood pressure 78/46 mmHg, and temperature 38° Celsius. A Swan-Ganz catheter was introduced and the following readings were obtained.

Central venous pressure (CVP) 8 mmHg   (ref 1– 7)
Pulmonary artery pressure   28/18 mmHg   (ref 15 - 25/8 - 15)
Pulmonary capillary wedge   15 mmHg   (ref 6 – 15)
pressure (PCWP)
Cardiac index (CI)   5.0 litre/min/m²   (ref 2.5 – 4.0)
Systemic vascular resistance   735 dynes/sec/cm⁻⁵/m²   (ref 1,500 – 3,000)
index (SVRI)
Pulmonary vascular resistance 150 dynes/sec/cm⁻⁵/m²   (ref 100 – 240)
index (PVRI)

Questions

1. What is the diagnosis?
2. List 5 other investigations.

Answers

1. Septic shock
2. Chest X-ray
   Blood cultures
   ECG
   Full blood count
   Renal, bone and liver chemistry profiles

Shock is a state of circulatory insufficiency leading to hypoperfusion and multiorgan failure. Shock can be due to:

- Cardiac causes (myocardial infarction, cardiac tamponade)
- Hypovolaemia (acute bleeding, dehydration)
- Sepsis
- Overdose
- Anaphylaxis

Patients often present with tachycardia, hypotension, confusion and oliguria. The systemic manifestations depend on the vital organs affected:

- CNS (confusion, drowsiness, coma)
- CVS (tachycardia, hypotension)
- Renal (oliguria)
- Skin (cold extremities, cyanosis)
- Systemic (pyrexia)

A combination of hypotension and metabolic acidosis points towards shock. Acidosis occurs due to the development of lactic acidosis secondary to hypoxia. The following indices measured with a Swan-Ganz catheter help to indicate the cause of shock.

	CO	SVRI	CVP	PCWP
Hypovolaemia	⇓	⇑	⇓	⇓
Cardiogenic	⇓	⇑	⇑	⇑
Sepsis	⇓	⇓	N/⇓	N/⇓

Key: CO = cardiac output; SVRI = systemic vascular resistance index; CVP = central venous pressure; PCWP = pulmonary capillary wedge pressure; ⇓ = decreased; ⇑ = increased; N = normal.

CASE 12

A 65-year-old lady was noted to have a cardiac murmur since childhood. She also had angina pectoris. At cardiac catheterisation the right coronary artery showed a proximal 50% stenosis, but the left coronary system was normal. The following haemodynamic data were obtained:

Right atrial pressure	8 mmHg ('v wave')
Right ventricular end-diastolic pressure	5 mmHg
Pulmonary artery pressure	72/32 mmHg
Pulmonary capillary wedge pressure	30 mmHg
Left ventricular end-diastolic pressure	12 mmHg

Question

What is the diagnosis?

Answer

The diagnosis is mitral stenosis. Note the higher pulmonary capillary wedge pressure compared to the left ventricular end-diastolic pressure.

Mitral Stenosis

This valvular disorder is almost invariably the delayed consequence of rheumatic heart disease, although a history of rheumatic fever in childhood is often absent. Less common causes of mitral stenosis are systemic lupus erythematosus, rheumatoid arthritis and congenital disorder. After rheumatic fever there is a latent period of 10-20 years before the onset of symptoms. In developed countries, rheumatic mitral stenosis presents in the third and fourth decade with symptoms of exertional dyspnoea, orthopnoea, paroxysmal nocturnal dyspnoea, which may be precipitated by the new onset of atrial fibrillation or pregnancy.

The clinical signs include a malar flush (mitral facies), a loud first heart sound, usually an opening snap, and an apical rumbling diastolic murmur. The ECG shows bifid P waves (P mitrale), unless there is atrial fibrillation. Echocardiography confirms the diagnosis and quantitates the severity of the lesion. The normal mitral valve area is 5 cm². When the valve area is less than 2 cm², a rise in left atrial pressure is inevitable, leading in turn to pulmonary venous hypertension, then pulmonary arterial hypertension, and ultimately right heart failure.

The treatment is warfarin to prevent thromboembolic complications, digoxin for control of atrial fibrillation, diuretics for pulmonary congestion, and antibiotic prophylaxis against bacterial endocarditis. Balloon valvuloplasty via a transatrial septal puncture is useful in young patients without calcified valves, particularly pregnant women, and other patients deemed unfit for mitral valve replacement. Contraindications to balloon valvuloplasty are mitral regurgitation and thrombus in the atrial appendage (visualised beforehand by transoesophageal echocardiography). Complications of valvuloplasty are pericardial tamponade due to perforation of the left atrium, systemic embolism of undetected atrial thrombus, induction of ventricular arrhythmias by the catheter, and mitral regurgitation after balloon dilatation. Restenosis could be as high as 50% of patients at 2 years.

Lutembacher syndrome is the combination of mitral stenosis and a left-to-right shunt at the atrium. This shunt could be due to a congenital atrial septal defect of the ostium secundum variety, or acquired as a complication of mitral valvuloplasty.

Prevention of Endocarditis in Adults

The British Heart Foundation in the UK encourages patients to carry an 'endocarditis dental warning card'. The following guidelines are taken from the British National Formulary (see www.bnf.org.uk).

Dental Procedures Under Local or no Anaesthetic

Dental procedures such as tooth extraction, scaling, or periodontal surgery require antibiotic prophylaxis.

Patients who have not received more than a single dose of penicillin in the previous month, including those with a prosthetic valve (but not those who have had endocarditis):

- single dose of amoxicillin 3 gram orally 1 hour before procedure

If allergic to penicillin or if penicillin has been taken more than once in the previous month:

- clindamycin 600 mg orally 1 hour before procedure

Patients who have had endocarditis, amoxicillin + gentamicin, as under general anaesthesia.

Dental Procedures under General Anaesthetic

No special risk:

- IV amoxicillin 1 gram at induction, then oral amoxicillin 500 mg 6 hours later.
- Or oral amoxicillin 3 gram 4 hours before induction then oral amoxicillin 3 gram as soon as possible after procedure.

Special risk (patients with prosthetic valve or who have had endocarditis):

- IV amoxicillin 1 gram + IV gentamicin 120 mg at induction, then oral amoxicillin 500 mg 6 hours later.

If allergic to pencillin or who have had more than one dose of penicillin in the previous month:

- IV vancomycin 1 gram over at least 100 minutes then IV gentamicin 120 mg at induction or 15 minutes before procedure.
- Or, IV teicoplanin 400 mg + gentamicin 120 mg at induction or 15 minutes before procedure.
- Or, IV clindamycin 300 mg over at least 10 minutes at induction or 15 minutes before procedure then oral or IV clindamycin 150 mg 6 hours later.

Upper Respiratory Procedures

As for dental procedures; postoperative dose may be given parenterally if swallowing is painful.

Genitourinary Procedures

As for special risk patients undergoing dental procedures under general anaesthetic except clindamycin is not given, see above; if urine infected, prophylaxis should cover infective organism.

Obstetric, Gynaecological and Gastrointestinal Procedures

Prophylaxis required for patients with prosthetic valve or those who have had endocarditis only, as for genitourinary procedures.

CASE 13

A 64-year-old man was admitted to the CCU with an acute inferior myocardial infarction. He was given diamorphine, oxygen, and streptokinase. Ten hours later he suddenly became hypotensive with a systolic blood pressure of 78 mmHg recorded by palpation and a regular heart rate of 92 bpm. The jugular venous pressure was elevated, but the chest was clear on auscultation.

Questions
1. What is the most likely diagnosis?
2. What two other investigations should have been done prior to the Swan-Ganz catheterisation?

Answers

1. Right ventricular infarction complicating acute inferior myocardial infarction
2. Electrocardiogram with right sided precordial leads and echocardiography

The right coronary artery supplies the right ventricle, inferobasal wall of the left ventricle, posterobasal parts of the left ventricle, and the inferior third of the interventricular septum. Right ventricular infarction (RVI) occurs if there is proximal occlusion of the right coronary artery. There is haemodynamic evidence of right ventricular dysfunction in 19 - 43% of patients with acute inferior myocardial infarction, but only 3 - 8% of these patients have clinical features of right ventricular dysfunction. These features are hypotension, which is due to the inability of the damaged right ventricle to maintain the filling of the left ventricle, and an elevated jugular venous pressure. Furthermore, the finding of clear lung fields and hypotension in the setting of an acute inferior myocardial infarction should always raise the suspicion of RVI.

When RVI is suspected the right sided precordial ECG leads should be recorded. The leads V3R and V4R may show Q waves and ST segment elevation of > 0.5 mm. Echocardiography shows inferior wall hypokinesia or akinesia with similar abnormalities of the right ventricular free wall and a dilated right ventricular cavity. The *normal* haemodynamic data of the right side of the heart are:

Right atrium (mean)	1-8 mmHg
Right ventricle (systolic)	15-28 mmHg
Right ventricle (end-diastole)	0-8 mmHg
Pulmonary artery (systolic)	15-25 mmHg
Pulmonary artery (end-diastole)	8-15 mmHg
Pulmonary artery (mean)	10-22 mmHg
Pulmonary capillary wedge pressure (mean)	6-15 mmHg

The essential haemodynamic findings of RVI are:
- Abnormally elevated right atrial pressure
- Elevated right ventricular pressures
- Increased ratio of right to left ventricular filling pressures

The differential diagnosis of RVI includes the following:
- Hypotension with acute left ventricular myocardial infarction
- Pericardial tamponade
- Constrictive pericarditis
- Pulmonary embolism

In RVI the mainstay of treatment is fluid therapy as guided by pulmonary wedge pressure, which is discontinued once it reaches 20-25 mmHg so as to avoid pulmonary oedema. Inotropes are needed when the blood pressure is not maintained despite optimal pulmonary wedge pressure.

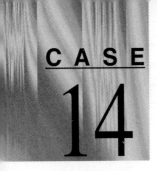

CASE 14

A 57-year-old man presented to the ENT department with hearing loss in the left ear. On examination, there was a left external squint and mild ataxia. An audiogram was arranged and the results are shown below.

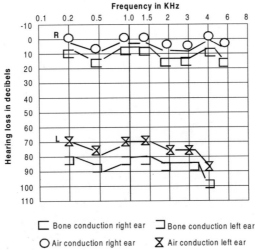

Frequency in KHz

	Bone conduction right ear		Bone conduction left ear
	Air conduction right ear		Air conduction left ear

Questions

1. What does the audiogram show?
2. What other investigation is essential to establish the diagnosis?

Answers

1. Left sensorineural deafness due to a cerebellopontine angle lesion such as acoustic neuroma or meningioma
2. MRI brain scan

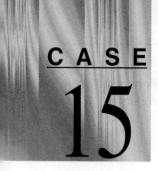

C A S E

15

CASE 15

A 35-year-old man presented to the Cardiology department with recurrent chest pains induced by exertion. M-mode echocardiogram showed the following:

Left ventricular dimensions		(normal range)
Interventricular septum at end-diastole	2.7 cm	(0.8 - 1.1)
Left ventricular posterior wall at end-diastole	1.5 cm	(0.5 - 1.1)
Left ventricular cavity internal dimension at end-diastole	2.5 cm	(2.5 - 4.5)

Questions
1. What is the echocardiographic diagnosis?
2. What other abnormalities are expected?

Answers

1. Hypertrophic cardiomyopathy (HCM).
2. Important echocardiographic features of hypertrophic cardiomyopathy include:

- Asymmetrical septal hypertrophy (ASH), which is present if the ratio of the interventricular septum to the posterior wall is > 1.5 in end-diastole.
- Systolic anterior motion of the mitral valve (SAM), which may not be seen at rest, but can be provoked by isovolumic exercises or Valsalva manoeuvre.
- Mid-systolic aortic valve closure and fluttering.

Asymmetrical septal hypertrophy occurs in about 60% of patients with hypertrophic cardiomyopathy, but there are other subtypes of left ventricular hypertrophy, including:

- Concentric hypertrophy (30%)
- Apical hypertrophy (10%)

However, neither SAM nor ASH is specific for hypertrophic cardiomyopathy. The former may occur in aortic stenosis, while the latter may be seen in mitral valve prolapse.

Continuous Wave Doppler can identify obstruction in the left ventricular outflow tract, which if present is below the level of a structurally normal aortic valve. If there is obstruction of the left ventricular outflow at a sub-valvular level, the condition is called hypertrophic obstructive cardiomyopathy (HOCM). Auscultation reveals an ejection systolic murmur similar to that of aortic stenosis.

About half of the patients with HCM have a positive family history and this condition is inherited as an autosomal dominant. The incidence of HCM is 0.4 - 2.5 per 100,000 of the population. The age of onset has a bimodal distribution with the first peak in the 2nd decade and a second peak during the 4th to 6th decades. Clinically it can be asymptomatic and present for the first time as sudden death due to ventricular fibrillation during exercise. Every year 3% of adults with HCM will succumb to Sudden Cardiac Death. Syncope or palpitation is due to a wide range of arrhythmias, including atrial or ventricular tachyarrhythmias, atrioventricular block, and sick sinus syndrome. Angina with normal coronary arteries is due to increased oxygen consumption caused by left ventricular hypertrophy. Heart failure is rare and produced by diastolic dysfunction and mitral regurgitation.

Treatment of HCM

- Implantable cardioverter defibrillator (ICD) for life threatening cardiac arrhythmias.
- Drugs, such as beta-blockers and amiodarone. Amiodarone is the only medication that has been shown to reduce sudden cardiac death.
- Left ventricular myomectomy
- Mitral valve replacement for regurgitation
- Right ventricular pacing pulls the septum away from the left ventricular outflow tract
- Catheter septal ablation. Ethanol (96%) is infused down the first septal branch of the left anterior descending artery and induces infarction of the proximal interventricular septum.

CASE 16

A 52-year-old man woke up one morning with weakness of the left arm and leg. He had been diabetic and hypertensive for the past 10 years. About five years earlier, he was treated for an acute myocardial infarction. His medications included glipizide, aspirin, ramipril and simvastatin. On examination, there was a left hemiparesis (power 3/5 in the arm and leg) and a right sided lower motor neurone facial palsy. The CT brain scan taken 48 hours later showed lacunar infarcts in the left basal ganglia.

Questions

1. Do the abnormalities on the CT brain scan explain the presenting neurological signs?
2. Where is the active lesion and what is the diagnosis?
3. What radiological investigation is likely to localise the lesion?

Answers

1. This patient presented with a sudden left hemiparesis while the CT scan has shown lacunar infarcts in the left basal ganglia. Therefore, the CT scan findings do not explain the presenting acute neurological deficit.
2. This patient has a right facial palsy of the lower motor neurone type and a 'crossed' left hemiparesis. This is called Millard-Gubler syndrome and the lesion is located in the right side of the pons.
3. MRI brain scan.

Brainstem Syndromes

The key features of brainstem syndromes are:

- Ipsilateral cranial nerve signs, i.e. on the same side as the lesion.
- Contralateral or 'crossed' hemiplegia, due to the involvement of the corticospinal tracts destined for the limbs on the opposite side of the body.
- The aetiology of these syndromes is usually a vascular lesion, i.e. occlusion of branches of the vertebral and basilar arteries, or tumour.

The following table describes some of the eponymous syndromes that present with contralateral or 'crossed' hemiplegia:

Eponym	Site of lesion	Cranial nerve affected	Major Neurological Signs
• Parinaud	High Midbrain		Paralysis of upward gaze & accommodation Retraction nystagmus Pupillary areflexia
• Weber	Midbrain	III	Ipsilateral oculomotor palsy + contralateral hemiplegia
• Benedict	Midbrain	III	Ipsilateral oculomotor palsy + contralateral ataxia and rubral tremor (due to involvement of the superior cerebral peduncle and red nucleus) + contralateral hemiplegia
• Millard-Gubler	Pons	VII +/- VI	Ipsilateral facial palsy + contralateral hemiplegia
• Foville	Pons	VII	Ipsilateral facial palsy + conjugate lateral gaze palsy (to side of lesion)

Contd...

Contd...

Eponym	Site of lesion	Cranial nerve affected	Major Neurological Signs
• Avellis	Medulla	X	Ipsilateral paralysis of palate & vocal cord + contralateral hemianaesthesia (spinothalamic) + contralateral hemiplegia
• Jackson	Medulla	X, XI, XII	Ipsilateral paralysis of palate & vocal cord Ipsilateral weakness of sternomastoid & trapezius Ipsilateral weakness of tongue + contralateral hemiplegia
• Wallenberg	Medulla + adjacent parts of cerebellum	Spinal nucleus of V, IX, X	Ipsilateral facial pain & temperature sensory loss Ipsilateral paralysis of palate & vocal cord
	+ Spinothalamic tracts		Ipsilateral ataxia & nystagmus Ipsilateral Horner's syndrome + contralateral spinothalamic sensory loss + contralateral hemiparesis (mild)

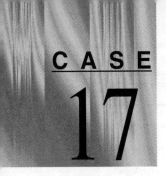

C A S E

17

CASE 17

A 76-year-old man presented to the Medical Assessment Unit with a history of collapse and was found to be confused. He had been attending his General Practitioner for abdominal pain. The biochemistry results were as follows:

Na	124 mmol/l
K	2.9 mmol/l
Urea	28 mmol/l
Glucose	5.7 mmol/l
HCO_3	45 mmol/l
Chloride	82 mmol/l

Questions
1. What are the metabolic abnormalities?
2. What is the most likely cause?

Answers

1. The patient has hyponatraemia and hypokalaemia, and the high urea indicates dehydration. The low chloride and high bicarbonate suggest he had repeated vomiting with resultant metabolic alkalosis.
2. The chronic abdominal pain and vomiting suggest pyloric stenosis

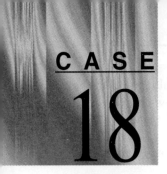

CASE 18

CASE 18

A 35-year-old man presented to the Cardiology department with shortness of breath. He underwent left and right heart catheterisation. Comment on the following data:

Chamber	Pressure (mmHg)	Oxygen Saturation (%)
Aorta	110/58	85
Left ventricle	110/58	85
Right atrium	12	68
Right ventricle	100/10	80
Pulmonary artery	100/72	80
Pulmonary capillary wedge	12	97

Question
1. What is the diagnosis?

Answer

Ventricular septal defect with Eisenmenger syndrome. Note the step-up of oxygen saturation at the level of the right ventricle indicating the site of the shunt. However, there is also severe pulmonary hypertension, which has caused reversal of the shunt leading to systemic oxygen desaturation, while the pulmonary venous blood at the level of the pulmonary wedge is fully saturated.

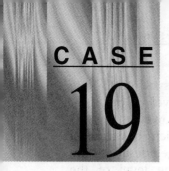

C A S E
19

CASE 19

Comment on the following data:

Albumin	44 g/l
Calcium	2.44 mmol/l
Corrected calcium	2.36 mmol/l
PO$_4$	2.28 mmol/l
ALP	289 U/l

Answer

This patient has marked hyperphosphataemia due to renal failure. The raised alkaline phosphatase indicates associated metabolic bone disease, which is initially osteomalacia. Secondary hyperparathyroidism in patients with renal failure may restore the serum calcium level to normal, as in this patient. PTH secretion eventually becomes autonomous, which is called tertiary hyperparathyroidism, and is characterised by hypercalcaemia.

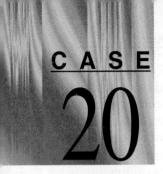

C A S E
20

CASE 20

A 44-year-old engineer from the Middle East presented with chronic shortness of breath. He had a resting tachycardia (96 bpm) and became easily tired on exercise. The jugular venous pressure was raised and a third heart sound was heard. Comment on the following pressure values obtained at cardiac catheterisation:

Right atrium	'a' wave 16 mmHg and 'v' wave 15 mmHg
Right ventricle	40/14 mmHg
Pulmonary artery	44/14 mmHg
Pulmonary artery wedge	14 mmHg (mean)

Question
1. What is the diagnosis?

Answer

The most likely diagnosis is constrictive pericarditis. Indeed, re-examination of the chest X-ray confirmed that pericardial calcification had been overlooked. The equalisation of the filling pressures is also seen in patients with cardiac tamponade. The following table summarises the differences and similarities between these two conditions:

	Cardiac tamponade	Constrictive pericarditis
• Jugular venous pressure	Prominent 'x' descent	Prominent 'x' and 'y' descent
• Kussmaul's sign	Usually absent	May be present
• Pulsus paradoxicus	Invariable	Not common
• Atrial pressures	Equal	Equal
• Left and right ventricular End-diastolic pressures	Equal	Equal
• Diastolic dip and plateau waveform §	Absent	Present

§ This is due to rapid ventricular filling followed by diastasis.

Clinically, differentiation of constrictive pericarditis and restrictive cardiomyopathy (e.g. amyloid disease) may be difficult. Both conditions may show:

1. Raised jugular venous pressure with prominent 'x' and 'y' descents
2. Normal systolic function
3. Diastolic dip and plateau waveform

However, in constrictive pericarditis the left and right ventricular end-diastolic pressures are equal. In restrictive cardiomyopathy they are different by at least > 7 mmHg, especially at the end of expiration.

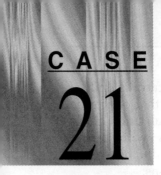

C A S E

21

CASE 21

An 80-year-old lady presented with confusion, abdominal pain and constipation. Routine blood tests revealed the following values:

Corrected calcium	3.11 mmol/l
PO_4	0.86 mmol/l
Bilirubin	10 µmol/l
ALT	39 U/l
ALP	75 U/l

Questions
1. Comment on the above results.
2. Give three common differential diagnoses.

Answers
1. Hypercalcaemia with low serum phosphate
2. Primary hyperparathyroidism
   Bony metastasis
   Multiple myeloma

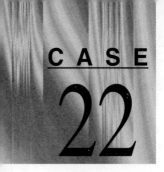

C A S E
22

CASE 22

A 75-year-old man presented with recurrent falls. He had been living alone over the last one year and had not been able to look after himself. Examination revealed a mask-like face and cogwheel rigidity in the upper limbs. During his stay in hospital the staff nurse reported that at night time he suffered from visual hallucinations, which were associated with restlessness and aggressiveness. His blood test results were as follows:

Hb	12.0 g/dl
WBC	$7.3 \times 10^9/l$
Platelets	$250 \times 10^9/l$
MCV	83 fl
Na	137 mmol/l
K	3.8 mmol/l
Urea	7.0 mmol/l
Creatinine	95 µmol/l
Bilirubin	10 µmol/l
ALT	100 U/l
ALP	35 U/l
Total protein	60 g/l
Albumin	40 g/l
Globulin	20 g/l
Corrected calcium	2.35 mmol/l
CRP	< 8 mg/l
Glucose	6.0 mmol/ l
TSH	1.25 mU/l

Question
1. What is the most likely diagnosis?

Answers

The diagnosis is Lewy body dementia.

Dementia is characterised by the progressive decline of mental abilities accompanied by changes in personality and behaviour. There is commonly a loss of memory and skills that are needed to carry out everyday activities. In the UK population an estimated 5% of those over the age of 65 have dementia and rising to 20% over the age of 80. The most common form of dementia is Alzheimer's disease (AD), which has characteristic histopathological features such as neurofibrillary tangles of paired helical filaments and amyloid plaques. About 50% of all dementia is due to AD. Vascular dementia or Multi-infarct dementia (MID) is characterised by the stepwise progression of the illness, the presence of vascular risk factors, and focal neurological signs. Neuroimaging in MID shows multiple cerebral infarcts. MID and AD can co-exist in about one third of patients with dementia.

Lewy Body Dementia

Lewy body dementia (LBD) is the second most common form of dementia and accounts for 15 to 25% of all cases. The average age of onset is 50–80 years and is commoner in men than women. LBD is suggested by the combination of impaired cognition, spontaneous parkinsonian features, and visual hallucinations, but memory function can be relatively well preserved in the early stages. Neuroimaging shows significantly greater medial temporal lobe (hippocampal) atrophy in LBD compared with AD and MID. Lewy bodies contain a presynaptic protein called alpha synuclein, which is targeted for removal by ubiquitin. Accumulation of alpha synuclein in brain cells could be due to the failure of enzymatic degradation.

Rapid eye movement (REM) sleep disturbance may be an early feature of LBD, but also occurs in Parkinson's disease and Multiple System Atrophy. In this condition REM motor atonia is partially or completely absent. People with this disorder are, therefore, able to move their muscles and act out their dreams. REM sleep disordered behaviour includes punching and kicking. Myoclonus is another common early presentation in LBD and may be confused with Creutzfeld-Jakob disease.

Neuroleptic treatment for hallucinations and other neuropsychiatric manifestations may worsen the parkinsonian features of LBD. In about half of all patients with LBD, deterioration in cognitive function, drowsiness and worsening parkinsonism can occur within 2 weeks of starting neuroleptic medication or a dose change. Hallucinations and delusion may respond better to one of the new antipsychotic drugs, such as clozapine and olanzapine, with less deterioration in Parkinsonism. L-dopa is used to treat the parkinsonian features, but may in turn aggravate confusion, hallucinations or delusions. Selegiline and anticholinergic agents are even less well tolerated. Low levels of acetylcholine can be shown in the brains of patients with LBD and anecdotal experience with acetylcholinesterase inhibitors, such as donepezil and rivastigmine, shows promising results in the control of neuropsychiatric symptoms. There is no cure for LBD and the condition is progressive, with a duration of illness of about 6 years.

Acetylcholinesterase Inhibitors in AD

Progressive loss of cholinergic neurons and impaired cholinergic transmission can be shown in the brains of patients with Alzheimer's disease. Acetylcholinesterase inhibitors restore acetylcholine levels by inhibiting its breakdown. In the UK, three acetylcholinesterase inhibitors (donepezil, rivastigmine, and galantamine) are licensed for use in patients with AD who have a MMSE score of 12 or more. The effect of these drugs is an improvement in the MMSE score of 1-2 points at 6 months, compared with an expected decline of 4-5 points at one year in patients given placebo. Improvements in behavioural symptoms, such as a reduction in agitation and aggression, and the delay in the need for nursing home placements by about 6 months appear promising. These drugs are currently not licensed for use in other forms of dementia.

The Folstein's Mini-mental Screening Examination (MMSE)

The MMSE is used to identify impaired cognition and documenting subsequent decline. Various aspects of cognition, such as orientation, concentration, memory and language abilities are evaluated and points are scored against each component.

The Clock Drawing Test

Asking the patient to draw a clock and set the time at 11:10 hours is a simple test of cognitive function. Failure to insert the correct numbers around the clock face and indicate the correct time can be scored using the method shown in the diagram on page 66.

Summary of Diagnostic Criteria for Common Forms of Dementia

Diagnostic Criteria for Alzheimer's disease (AD)
(from the Diagnostic and Statistical Manual of Mental Disorders, DSM-IV 1994)

- Memory impairment (i.e. inability to learn and recall new information).
- One or more of the following cognitive deficits: aphasia, apraxia, agnosia, impaired executive function (i.e. planning, sequential organisation, attention)
- Loss of social and occupational function due to cognitive failure
- Gradual onset and progressive cognitive decline
- Exclude other neurological diseases that impair cognition (e.g. strokes, hydrocephalus, subdural haematoma, Huntingtons's chorea, Parkinson's disease).
- Exclude systemic medical disorders that impair cognition (e.g. hypothyroidism, hypercalcaemia, syphilis, HIV, and deficiencies of vitamin B_{12}, folate, and niacin).
- Exclude cognitive failure secondary to drug abuse (e.g. sedatives, alcohol)
- Exclude other psychiatric conditions that impair cognition (e.g. depression or schizophrenia).
- Cognitive defects do not occur exclusively during delirium

Diagnostic criteria for vascular dementia (VD)
(from DSM-IV 1994)

- Presence of a dementia syndrome (i.e. poor memory and other cognitive deficits)

- Focal neurological signs and symptoms, or neuroimaging evidence of cerebrovascular disease, which are judged to be aetiologically relevant.
- Symptoms do not occur exclusively during delirium.

Diagnostic Criteria for Lewy Body Dementia (LBD)

(from Dementia with Lewy bodies international workshop: McKeith IG et al. Neurology 1996; 47: 1113-24.)

Two of the following = probable LBD.
One of the following = possible LBD.

- Fluctuating cognition with pronounced variation in attention and alertness
- Recurrent visual hallucinations (i.e. fully formed images of 3-dimensional objects, people, or animals).
- Spontaneous motor features of Parkinsonism

Clinical features that are supportive of LBD are:
- Repeated falls
- Syncope or transient loss of consciousness
- Neuroleptic sensitivity
- Systemised delusions (e.g. false belief that there are strangers in the house; deceased friends or relatives are visiting).
- Hallucinations in other modalities (e.g. auditory hallucinations include banging, knocking, footsteps, or muffled voices).

Differential Diagnosis of Different Forms of Dementia

	Lewy Body Dementia	Alzheimer's Disease	Vascular Dementia
• Onset	variable	gradual	relatively sudden
• Cognition at onset	may be 'normal'	impaired	impaired
• Fluctuation in cognition	early and sustained	rare	markedly at night ('sundowners')
• Progress of illness	variable	gradual	step-wise

N.B. The clinical diagnostic accuracy of the type of dementia is 71% to 88%. Patients could have mixed pathology, e.g. cerebrovascular disease and therefore vascular dementia, as well as Alzheimer's disease.

The Folstein Mini-mental State Examination (MMSE)*

	COMPONENTS	POINTS
	Orientation	
1	Year	1
	Season	1
	Date	1
	Day	1
	Month	1
2	Name of building	1
	Floor	1
	Town	1
	County	1
	Country	1
	Registration	
3	Name three objects and ask patient to repeat all three. E.g. 'Ball, Flag, Chair'. Repeat until patient can correctly name all three objects.	3
	Attention and calculation	
4	Spell the word ' WORLD' backwards	5
	Recall	
5	Ask name of three objects said earlier	3
	Language	
6	Ask patient to name two objects (e.g. pencil and watch)	2
7	Ask patient to repeat 'No ifs, ands, or buts'	1
8	Ask patient to follow a three-stage command: 'Take the paper in your right hand. Fold the paper in half. Put the paper on the floor.'	3
9	Ask patient to read and obey a command: 'Close your eyes.'	1
10	Ask patient write a full sentence	1
11	Ask patient to copy a design	1

* Folstein MF, Folstein SE & McHugh PR. Mini-Mental State: A practical method for grading the cognitive state of patients for the clinician. Journal of Psychiatric Research 1975; 12:189-198.

N.B. MMSE scores of less than 24 are generally considered to be abnormal. However, there is an inverse relationship between MMSE scores and age. The median score is 29 for 18-24 year olds. The median score is 25 for individuals over the age of 80 years. MMSE scores are also adversely affected by poor educational attainment, poor vision, language difficulties, depression, and delirium. In the UK National Institute of Clinical Excellence (NICE) 2001 guidelines:

• MMSE scores of 21-26 suggest mild dementia.

- MMSE scores of 10-20 suggest moderate dementia
- MMSE scores of less than 10 suggest severe dementia

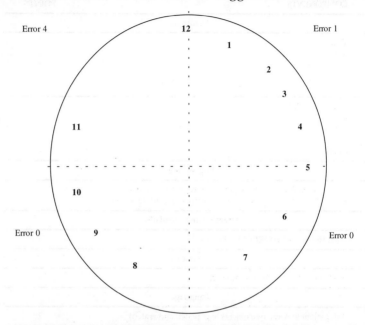

The Clock Drawing Test
(Agrell and Dehlin, Age and Ageing 1998;27:399-403)

Watson's score for the Clock Drawing Test

1. Draw the first reference line between the centre & the number 12.
   Draw the second line perpendicular to it.
2. Count the number of digits in each quadrant.
   If a digit falls on a reference line, it is included in the next quadrant.
3. Three digits per quadrant are correct.
   An error score of 1 is assigned for mistakes in each of the first *three* quadrants.
   An error score of 4 is assigned for the *fourth* quadrant.
Normal range = scores 0 – 3
Score of 4 or more is abnormal
Maximum score = 7
In the example below, the total error score is = 5

CASE 23

A 60-year-old man was admitted with a vertebral fracture. There was no significant past medical history apart from a history of mumps as a child. He was married with no children. Bone mineral density was measured with the results shown below:

	Bone Mineral Density (BMD)	Result expressed as % of a young adult's BMD		Result expressed as % of age & sex matched subject's BMD	
		%	T	%	Z
Lumbar spine L1	0.773 g/cm²	67	-3.23	69	-2.88
Lumbar spine L2	0.867 g/cm²	70	-3.11	72	-2.76
Femoral neck	0.857 g/cm²	80	-1.64	90	-0.71

Questions
1. What do the results show?
2. What other investigations would you consider in this individual?

Answers

1. Osteoporosis of L1 and L2 vertebrae.
2. Serum testosterone levels.

Osteoporosis is characterised by a low bone mass or density resulting in an increased risk of fracture. Osteoporosis is usually primary (idiopathic) and a secondary cause is more often encountered in men than women, including:
- Prolonged oral corticosteroid use
- Hypogonadism
- Hyperparathyroidism
- Hyperthyroidism
- Alcohol abuse
- Anticonvulsants
- Multiple myeloma
- Bony metastasis

Osteoporosis is diagnosed in the presence of one of the following:
- A history of low velocity trauma fracture.
- A low bone mineral density (BMD), which is measured by dual energy X-ray absorptiometry (DEXA).

The World Health Organisation (WHO) has defined osteoporosis as a BMD of 2.5 standard deviations or more below the mean value for young adults (T score less than - 2.5), whereas a T score value between - 1.0 and - 2.5 represents osteopenia. There is a strong link between low BMD and an increased risk of fracture. However, screening the general population for low BMD is not advocated, as there is no evidence that this strategy reduces the risk of fractures. The Royal College of Physicians (RCP) in the UK has recommended measuring BMD in selected groups of patients, such as:
- X-ray evidence of osteopenia or osteoporosis.
- Previous low velocity trauma fracture
- Premature menopause (age < 45 years)
- Prolonged secondary amenorrhoea
- Prolonged oral corticosteroid use (equivalent to more than 7.5 mg a daily of prednisolone for 6 months or longer)
- Primary hypogonadism
- Maternal history of hip fracture

- Chronic disorders associated with an increased risk of osteoporosis (e.g. coeliac disease, chronic liver disease, hyperthyroidism, hyperparathyroidism)
- Low body mass index (BMI < 19)

Management includes

- Appropriate investigations (ESR and full blood count; renal, bone, and liver chemistry profiles; serum electrophoresis; prostate specific antigen; thyroid function, testosterone, luteinising hormone, follicle stimulating hormone, and sex hormone binding globulin).
- Advice on life style measures (regular exercise, balanced diet rich in calcium, reduced alcohol consumption).
- Drugs (calcium and vitamin D, bisphosphonates, calcitonin, recombinant human parathyroid hormone, and testosterone in hypogonadal men. In women hormone replacement therapy is available for the prophylaxis of postmenopausal osteoporosis. An alternative is raloxifene, which is used for both the prevention and treatment of postmenopausal osteoporosis).

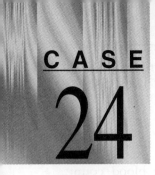

CASE 24

An 87-year-old woman presented with painful micturition and macroscopic haematuria. She was a life long non-smoker with no previous hospital admissions. Her medications were atenolol for hypertension and co-amilofruse for dependent oedema. Physical examination was unremarkable.

Hb	12.5 g/dl
WBC	12.9 x 10^9/l
Platelets	420 x 10^9/l
INR	1.1
Na	136 mmol/l
K	3.9 mmol/l
Urea	16.7 mmol/l
Creatinine	158 µmol/l
Albumin	36 g/l
Globulin	44 g/l
Bilirubin	8 µmol/l
ALP	116 U/l
ALT	16 U/l
TSH	3.07 mU/l
Corrected calcium	3.18 mmol/l
Protein electrophoresis	no monoclonal bands
Bence-Jones protein	negative
PTH	< 0.1 pmol/l
PTH-rP	10 pmol/l (ref < 2.6)
MSU	no growth
CXR	normal
Isotope bone scan	normal
CT abdomen	bladder tumour with bilateral hydronephrosis
Cystoscopic biopsy	poorly differentiated transitional cell carcinoma of the bladder

Questions
1. What is the cause of her hypercalcaemia?
2. What is the treatment?

Answers

1. Hypercalcaemia in malignancy may be due to metastatic disease, or humoral substances such as PTH-rP, 1,25 hydroxyvitamin D, and prostaglandins. Hypercalcaemia in bladder cancer is very rare with a reported rate of 1.9% in a series of 321 cases. In this patient the hypercalcaemia was due to parathyroid hormone-related peptide (PTH-rP) production from a transitional cell bladder tumour. The human PTH-rP gene is located on the short arm of chromosome 12, and the human PTH gene is located on the short arm of chromosome 11. PTH-rP is structurally similar to PTH, and has the same affinity for PTH receptors in bone and kidney. Therefore, the hypercalcaemic effects of PTH-rP and PTH are similar, including:
   * increased renal calcium absorption
   * bone resorption
   * increased renal synthesis of 1,25 hydroxyvitamin D
2. Hypercalcaemia in malignancy may respond to:
   * IV normal saline and IV furosemide restore glomerular function and stimulate sodium-linked calcium diuresis in the proximal renal tubule. Remember to stop any medication that encourages calcium retention, e.g. thiazide diuretics.
   * IV pamidronate, IV or oral clodronate. Both bisphosphonates inhibit bone resorption.
   * Corticosteroids
   * Calcitonin
   * Chemotherapy
   * Dialysis

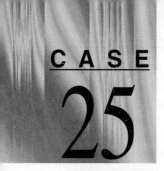

C A S E

25

CASE 25

A 31-year-old woman was admitted with a 7 days history of flu-like symptoms, fever, headache and vomiting. She was 4 weeks post-partum and had taken ibuprofen for a painful episiotomy wound. On examination, the pulse was 80 bpm regular, BP 120/55 mmHg, temperature 37° Celsius. There was no photophobia or nuchal rigidity and Kernig's sign was negative. Neurological examination including optic fundi was normal. The next day her temperature rose to 38.7° Celsius and there was definite nuchal rigidity. A lumbar puncture was performed (see results below). No treatment was given and over the next 10 days her temperature returned to normal. She made a complete recovery.

Hb	12.0 g/dl
WBC	8.3 x 10⁹/l (normal differential)
Platelets	270 x 10⁹/l
CRP	< 10 mg/l
U & E	normal
LFT	normal
Urinalysis	normal
CXR	normal
CT brain scan	normal
CSF pressure	20 cm
CSF appearance	clear and colourless; no organisms seen on microscopy
CSF white cells	170/ml (95% lymphocytes)
CSF red cells	30/ml
CSF protein	1.1 g/l
CSF glucose	2.9 mmol/l (blood glucose 5.3 mmol/l)
CSF culture	negative

Questions
1. What is the most likely diagnosis?
2. What are the possible causes?
3. What further investigations are required?

Answers

1. Lymphocytic meningitis
The presence of large numbers of lymphocytes in the CSF without evidence of bacterial infection is referred to as lymphocytic meningitis or aseptic meningitis. Lymphocytic meningitis is usually of viral aetiology, but there are many non-infective causes. The polymerase chain reaction (PCR), which can rapidly identify small amounts of viral and bacterial nucleic acid, has improved the diagnostic accuracy. However, an exact microbiological diagnosis is still only possible in about 10% of patients. If the patient is seriously ill and bacterial meningitis cannot be excluded on clinical grounds, IV cefotaxime and vancomycin should be given while waiting for microbiological confirmation. Similarly if viral encephalitis is suspected, IV acyclovir should be given.

2. The following conditions are associated with a predominantly lymphocytic picture in the CSF:

Infective

- Partially treated bacterial meningitis
- Viral meningitis: mumps, measles, polio, echo, coxsackie, cytomegalovirus, Epstein-Barr, herpes simplex, varicella zoster, HIV
- Brain abscess
- Sinus infection
- Non-pyogenic bacteria: TB, listeria, brucella, borrelia (Lyme's disease), treponema pallidum (syphilis), leptospira
- Fungal infection: candida, cryptococcus

Non-infective

- Leukaemia
- Lymphoma
- Sarcoidosis
- Systemic lupus erythematosus
- Cerebral venous sinus thrombosis
- Drugs (NSAID, aspirin, IV immunoglobulin, co-trimoxazole)

3. In this patient the following test results were obtained:

ESR	28 mm/h
Paul Bunnell	negative
Blood culture	negative
MSU culture	negative
CSF culture	negative
PCR of CSF	negative for mycobacterial antigen
CSF TB culture	negative
MRA	normal
Virus culture	throat swab, stool, CSF – all negative
Viral serology	negative
Syphilis serology	negative
Anti-DNA, RA latex	negative
CSF cytology	reactive lymphocytes

The remaining diagnostic possibility in this patient is ibuprofen induced aseptic lymphocytic meningitis.

CASE 26

A 75-year-old woman was admitted to hospital with a fracture of the left pubic ramus due to an accidental fall. Past medical history included myocardial infarction, chronic atrial fibrillation, left ventricular failure, and Parkinson's disease. Her medications were aspirin 75 mg od, furosemide 40 mg od, lisinopril 20 mg od, digoxin 62.5 µg od, Madopar CR 250 mg tds. Subcutaneous heparin 5,000 units twice daily was given to prevent thromboembolic disease. Ten days into her stay in hospital, she developed acute ischaemia of the left leg. Embolectomy was unsuccessful and she was prepared for a below knee amputation. Blood tests taken before surgery showed:

Hb	11.2 g/dl
WBC	9.7 x 10⁹/l
Platelets	46 x 10⁹/l
Prothrombin time	12 seconds

Questions
1. What is the diagnosis?
2. What is the treatment?

Answers

1. Heparin induced thrombocytopenia (HIT) with arterial thrombosis.

HIT occurs in about 5% of patients receiving standard ('unfractionated') heparin treatment, usually at the end of 5 to 15 days of therapy. In about 10-20% of patients with HIT, serious arterial thrombotic complications develop including lower limb gangrene, stroke, and myocardial infarction. The thrombotic process in HIT requires an IgG antibody that binds to heparin. This heparin-IgG complex then attaches itself to the Fc receptors located on platelet membranes and initiates platelet aggregation. Diagnostic confirmation of HIT comes from platelet aggregation studies, which also demonstrate whether the IgG antibody will cross-react with low molecular weight heparin.

2. The treatment of HIT includes:
- Stop the unfractionated heparin
- Consider alternative anticoagulants such as:
  - Warfarin
  - Low molecular weight heparin (e.g. tinzaparin), or heparinoid (e.g. danaparoid), or hirudin (e.g. lepirudin), if the platelet aggregation studies show no cross-reaction.
  - Ancrod is a defibrinogenating enzyme derived from the venom of the Malayan pit viper. Ancrod cleaves fibrinopeptide A from fibrinogen and rapidly depletes fibrinogen levels
  - Fibrinolytic agents: streptokinase, tPA
- Other measures to prevent pulmonary embolism, e.g. IVC filter.

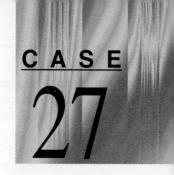
CASE 27

A 36-year-old mentally retarded woman who lived in a residential home was found unconscious at 08.00 hours and admitted to hospital. When assessed by her carers 12 hours earlier she had appeared to be well. Past psychiatric history included depression and behavioural problems with self inflicted injuries and self-poisoning from overdoses of paracetamol. She was treated for asthma and epilepsy. Her medications included temazepam 10 mg nocte, thioridazine 50 mg tds, procyclidine 10 mg tds, carbamazepine 400 mg bd, dosulepin 150 mg od, and salbutamol inhaler. On examination, her Glasgow Coma Scale was 7 (eye opening to pain = 2; flexion to pain = 3; verbal response = 2). Pulse 70 bpm regular, BP 110/70 mmHg, temperature 36° Celsius. There were no focal neurological signs or abnormalities in the chest, heart, and abdomen.

Na	137 mmol/l
K	4.1 mmol/l
Urea	2.4 mmol/l
HCO_3	19 mmol/l
Creatinine	60 µmol/l
Plasma glucose	0.1 mmol/l
Hb	13.3 g/dl
WBC	8.9 x 10^9/l
Platelets	370 x 10^9/l
CRP	< 8 mg/l
CXR	normal
Urinalysis	normal
Toxicology	negative for salicylates and paracetamol

Questions
1. What is the cause of this patient's coma?
2. What further investigations would you perform?

Answers

1. Hypoglycaemic coma
2. Other investigations, with results shown for this patient, would include:

- Plasma insulin = 49 mU/l (= 340 pmol/l)
- C-peptide = 1918 pmol/l
- Plasma glibenclamide = 54 µg/l (on admission) and 20 µg/l (after 28 hours)
- CT brain – normal
- CT pancreas – normal

In the UK drug or alcohol poisoning is the most common cause of coma and account for about 33-40% of cases presenting to casualty departments. Causes of coma can be easily recalled from the following aide-mémoire:

A = Apoplexy i.e. Stroke
E = Epilepsy
I = Injury, subdural haematoma, or tumour;
  Infections, meningitis or encephalitis
O = Overdose and alcohol intoxication
U = Uraemia and metabolic causes (e.g. hypoglycaemia, hyperglycaemia, hepatic failure, hypoxia, hyponatraemia, hypernatraemia)

This patient's hypoglycaemic coma was due to glibenclamide ingestion. Administration of all medications was supervised in this residential home, where one diabetic patient was taking glibenclamide regularly. Hence, she could have received glibenclamide accidentally. After taking a dose of glibenclamide the blood level of the drug peaks at about 200 µg/l and its elimination half life is about 12 hours. The glibenclamide level of 54 µg/l in this patient suggested ingestion of the drug at least 24 hours before.

During insulin release proinsulin is cleaved into C-peptide and insulin, both of which enter the circulation in equimolar amounts. Therefore, C-peptide provides information on insulin secretion. However, due to differences in metabolism the half-life of C-peptide is 30 minutes, compared with 5 minutes for insulin. This means C-peptide levels are about 5 times that of insulin. In this patient the C-peptide (pmol/l)/insulin (pmol/l) ratio of around 5 suggests endogenous insulin secretion. C-peptide levels are suppressed in response to exogenous insulin, but the levels are high in insulinoma and in response to sulphonylurea.

Hypoglycaemia

Hypoglycaemia may be fasting or reactive. Reactive or post-prandial hypoglycaemia may occur after gastric surgery. Non-specific symptoms in someone who has not had any previous gastric surgery may be incorrectly attributed to reactive hypoglycaemia on the basis of a prolonged glucose tolerance test (GTT). However, the prolonged GTT is unreliable as one third of normal subjects may develop hypoglycaemia with or without symptoms during the five hour test.

Fasting hypoglycaemia is arbitrarily defined as a plasma glucose of 2.5 mmol/l or less after an overnight fast. N.B. A plasma glucose of 2.5 mmol/l is equivalent to a blood glucose of 2.2 mmol/l. The speed of fall in blood sugar determines the probability of symptoms, which are either autonomic or cognitive. Epinephrine, growth hormone, and ACTH are released when plasma glucose is < 3.9 mmol/l. Generally speaking a plasma glucose of < 2.8 mmol/l will impair brain function. However, the plasma glucose threshold for triggering the onset of hypoglycaemic symptoms will change in an individual with frequent hypoglycaemia. This is because chronic hypoglycaemia leads to the up-regulation of the glucose transporter 1 protein (GLUT 1) at the blood-brain barrier.

Hypoglycaemic Symptoms

Autonomic symptoms are due to the activation of the sympathetic and parasympathetic nervous system in response to falling glucose:
- Sweating
- Palpitation ⎫
- Tremor ⎬ sympathetic
- Anxiety ⎭
- Hunger   (parasympathetic; leads to weight gain)

Cognitive symptoms are due to neuroglycopenia:
- Confusion
- Speech problems

- Headache
- Loss of concentration
- Amnesia
- Seizures
- Coma

Causes of Fasting Hypoglycaemia

- Insulinoma
  Insulinomas are rare pancreatic islet cell tumours that secrete insulin (see below).
- Liver failure
  The liver contains 100 gram of glycogen. Hepatic glucose output from glycogenolysis is approximately 7 mmol per minute and can maintain normal plasma glucose for several hours, but thereafter normoglycaemia requires gluconeogenesis.
- Alcohol inhibits gluconeogenesis. Hypoglycaemia can still occur when blood alcohol level is only half of the legal limit of 80 mg/dl.
- Addison's disease (cortisol facilitates gluconeogenesis).
- Hypopituitarism and hypothyroidism.
- Glycogen storage disease: fructose intolerance and galactosaemia.
- Insulin Growth Factor-2 (IGF-2) producing tumours, e.g. mesenchymal tumour, mesothelioma, fibrosarcoma, leiomyosarcoma, neurofibrosarcoma, hepatoma, adrenal carcinoma, lymphoma. IGF-2 stimulates peripheral glucose uptake and inhibit hepatic glucose output; insulin levels are < 8 μU/ml; IGF-2 tumours do not respond to diazoxide.
- Renal failure (hypoglycaemia is due to failure to clear insulin; uraemia also impairs gluconeogenesis).
- Insulin autoantibodies bind to insulin and lead to inappropriate insulin delivery and hypoglycaemia: associated with Graves' disease, Rheumatoid Arthritis, SLE, myelomatous paraproteinaemia, hydralazine and procainamide. Dissociation of the insulin-antibody immune complex releases free insulin and leads to hypoglycaemia.
- Insulin receptor antibodies occur in combination with insulin resistance, acanthosis nigricans, anti-DNA antibody, ANA, high gamma globulins and low serum complement.

Insulin receptor antibody can have both agonistic (i.e. hypoglycaemia inducing) and antagonistic (i.e. insulin-resistant diabetes producing) effects.

- Cardiac failure, malaria, disseminated malignancy.
- Drugs: beta blockers, ACE-I, aspirin, pentamidine (causes beta cell lysis), high dose co-trimoxazole.

Insulinoma

- Incidence 4 per million
- Can occur at any age
- 10% of these tumours are malignant.
- 10% are multiple
- 10% of cases form part of Multiple Endocrine Adenomatosis (MEA) type 1.
- Some patients do not harbour an insulinoma, but instead have diffuse islet cell hyperplasia, or nesidioblastosis (neodifferentiation of islet of Langerhans from pancreatic ducts).

Diagnostic Tests in Cases of Suspected Insulinoma

- 72-hour fast.
- Exclude sulphonylurea abuse.
- Hydroxybutyrate levels
- Pro-insulin and C-peptide levels
- Amended Insulin-Glucose ratio
- Failure of C-peptide suppression during IV insulin infusion.
- IV tolbutamide test
- Glucagon stimulation test

Hydroxybutyrate Levels

Excessive insulin release by sulphonylurea or insulinoma will suppress lipolysis and give rise to low fasting levels of hydroxybutyrate.

Proinsulin and C-peptide Levels

Proinsulin is measured using sensitive monoclonal antibodies. In normal subjects <20% of the total immunoreactive insulin is from proinsulin. In insulinoma, proinsulin levels are increased and make up >30% of total immunoreactive insulin.

The Amended Insulin-Glucose Ratio

In healthy subjects insulin secretion stops at a plasma glucose of around 1.7 mmol/l. The amended insulin-glucose ratio is used in the interpretation of insulin and glucose values taken during a prolonged fast:

$$\text{Amended insulin-glucose ratio} = \frac{\text{plasma insulin (mU/l or }\mu\text{U/ml)}}{\text{plasma glucose (mmol/l)} - 1.7}$$

In normal subjects the amended insulin-glucose ratio will be <10. In cases of proven insulinoma this ratio will be >30.

IV Insulin C-peptide Suppression Test

IV insulin (0.1 U/kg per hour) suppresses endogenous insulin secretion and C-peptide levels. A plasma glucose of < 2.5 mmol/l with an inappropriately high C-peptide level of > 0.2 nmol/l is suggestive of insulinoma.

IV Tolbutamide Test

This is reserved for patients when a 72 hour fast is inconclusive. In healthy subjects tolbutamide produces insulin release and a fall in blood sugar, both of which then returns to normal in about 3 hours. In insulinoma the drop in glucose and insulin release are much greater and prolonged.

- One gram tolbutamide in 20 ml of sterile water is given IV over 2 minutes.
- Insulin is measured every 5 minutes for 15 minutes
- Insulin level > 195 μU/ml suggests insulinoma
- Only half of insulinoma patients will have a positive tolbutamide response; also false positive results occur in obesity and liver disease
- Danger of prolonged and refractory hypoglycaemia.

Glucagon Stimulation Test

Glucagon causes a rise in glucose, which returns to normal in about 3 hours. In insulinoma the rise in glucose with glucagon is followed by an exaggerated insulin release and prolonged hypoglycaemia.

- One milligram of glucagon is given IV.
- Insulin is measured every 5 minutes for 15 minutes.

- Insulin level > 135 µU/ml suggests insulinoma.
- Only half of insulinoma patients will have a positive glucagon response.
- Danger of prolonged hypoglycaemia from massive insulin release.

Localisation of Insulinoma

- CT or MRI scan (80% of tumours are less than 2 cm, so a negative scan does not confidently exclude an insulinoma).
- Venous sampling for insulin
- Angiography.
- Octreotide scan.
- Pre-operative or intraoperative ultrasound is allegedly the best method.

Treatment of Insulinoma

- Surgery: glucose infusion during surgery, pre-operative diazoxide, post-operative hyperglycaemia may last for several days (from operative pancreatitis, and suppression of normal beta cell function by long standing hypoglycaemia).
- Diazoxide 100 mg tds inhibits insulin release (by stimulating alpha receptors on pancreatic beta cells) and promotes glycogenolysis (by inhibiting phosphodiesterase). Salt and water retention side effects can be counteracted by high dose thiazides.
- Verapamil inhibits insulin release in vitro. May be worth trying.
- Octreotide 50 µg s/c bd may be worth trying, but it has higher affinity for anterior pituitary somatostatin receptor-2 than the pancreatic somatostatin receptor-5.
- Streptozotocin for metastatic disease.

The 72-hour Fast

- Stop all non-essential medications.
- Calorie-free drink is provided; caffeine free.
- Physical activity is encouraged.
- Glucose, insulin, C-peptide, pro-insulin are measured 6 hourly.
- If glucose < 3.3 mmol/l, do the above blood tests hourly.

- End the fast if plasma glucose < 2.5 mmol/l and symptoms of hypoglycaemia, collect blood for glucose, insulin, C-peptide, pro-insulin, sulphonylurea metabolite, then give 1mg glucagon IV, re-measure glucose 10, 20, 30 minutes and then feed the patient.

Interpretation of the 72-hour Fast

	Normal subject	Insulinoma	Factitious Hypoglycaemia	Sulphonylurea induced hypoglycaemia
Hypoglycaemic symptoms & signs	No	Yes	Yes	Yes
Plasma glucose (mmol/l)	>2.5	< 2.5	< 2.5	<2.5
Plasma insulin (µU/ml)	<6	>6	>6	>6
C-peptide (nmol/l)	<0.2	>0.2	<0.2	>0.2
Proinsulin (pmol/l)	<5	>5	<5	>5
Hydroxybutyrate (nmol/l)	>2.7	<2.7	<2.7	<2.7
Presence of sulphonylurea or metabolite in blood	No	No	No	Yes

Guidance Notes on the 72-hour Fast

Insulin levels must be processed quickly: serum should be separated and frozen within 2 hours to prevent proteolytic breakdown of insulin. Insulin assays cannot distinguish between endogenous insulin and injected forms of human and animal insulins. Previous insulin treatment stimulates the production of antibodies that interfere with insulin assay.

In normal men plasma glucose does not fall below 3 mmol/l during a 72 hour fast. In some normal women, especially during pregnancy, plasma glucose may fall below 1.7 mmol/l, possibly due to fetal consumption, but this is not associated with symptoms, because ketosis provides fuel for brain function and the plasma insulin is suppressed to < 6 µU/ml.

CASE 28

A General Practitioner referred a 78-year-old woman to the Radiology Department for investigation of pain and swelling in the left calf. The venogram showed extensive venous thrombosis involving the left femoral, popliteal and calf veins. The chest X-ray was normal. She was started on s/c heparin and oral warfarin as an out-patient. Two months later she was sent into hospital with acute breathlessness. On admission her INR was 1.7 and a ventilation perfusion lung scan confirmed multiple pulmonary emboli. She was restarted on heparin while the warfarin dose was readjusted. After discharge from hospital the INR was carefully monitored and maintained between 2 and 3. Three weeks after leaving hospital she was readmitted with right sided pleuritic chest pain, haemoptysis and painful swelling of the right leg. During this second admission an enlarged lymph node was found above the left clavicle. The following results became available:

Hb	13.0 g/dl
WBC	13.0 x 10^9/l
Platelets	306 x 10^9/l
INR	2.6
U & E	normal
ALP	181 U/l
CXR	shadowing in the lower lobes of both lungs

Questions
1. What other investigations would you ask for?
2. How would you manage this patient?

Answers

1. The following investigations and results were obtained:
   - Venogram showed an extensive DVT in the right leg.
   - CT chest showed an embolus in the main pulmonary artery, mediastinal lymphadenopathy and lymphangitis.
   - Fine needle aspiration-biopsy of the left supraclavicular lymph node showed a metastatic adenocarcinoma.
   - Barium meal showed a stricture at the gastro-oesophageal junction. She was too unwell to have an endoscopic examination and biopsy.
   - Ultrasound of the abdomen and pelvis was normal.
2. The therapeutic options would include IVC filter and IV heparin.

This elderly patient developed extensive venous thrombosis in both lower limbs with pulmonary embolism despite warfarin treatment. This should lead to a careful search for an underlying "acquired or secondary" disorder associated with thrombophilia (or hypercoagulability). A congenital/genetic thrombophilic disorder would be unlikely to manifest for the first time so late in life.

Acquired or Secondary Causes of Thrombophilia

Virchow's triad describes the 3 groups of conditions that predispose to venous thrombosis: vessel wall injury, abnormal blood flow, and disorders in blood composition. In view of the overlap between vessel damage and altered blood flow, acquired hypercoagulability can be simply divided into two groups:

Disorders in Blood Vessels and Blood Flow

- Immobilisation
- Trauma and surgery
- Obesity
- Indwelling central venous catheters
- Hyperviscosity syndromes: Waldenström's macroglobulinaemia, multiple myeloma
- Vasculitis

- Hyperhomocysteinaemia causes endothelial damage, platelet activation, and thrombosis.
  N.B. Secondary causes of hyperhomocysteinaemia include: nutritional deficiencies (folate, vitamin B_{12} and pyridoxine), diabetes mellitus, smoking, renal failure, hypothyroidism, cancer (especially breast and pancreas).

Disorders in Coagulation

- Malignancy with or without disseminated intravascular coagulation
- Nephrotic syndrome
- Lupus anticoagulant/antiphospholipid syndrome
- Oestrogens and the oral contraceptive pill
- L-asparaginase treatment
- Myeloproliferative disease: polycythaemia vera, essential thrombocythaemia
- Paroxysmal nocturnal haemoglobinuria
- Heparin induced thrombocytopenia
- Thrombotic thrombocytopenic purpura

Malignant tumours promote thromboembolic disease by activation of factor VII in the extrinsic coagulation pathway and factor XII in the intrinsic coagulation pathway. Heparin inhibits factor VII and may be more effective if there is failure to control thrombotic disease despite therapeutic doses of warfarin in patients with malignancy. Tumours that are associated with thrombotic disease include:

- Gastrointestinal cancer: in one series colorectal, gastric, and pancreatic cancer accounted for 67% of cases.
- Gynaecological cancer (15%)
- Breast cancer (9%)

Testing for Genetic Causes of Thrombophilia

If there is no obvious secondary cause for venous thrombosis, the following clinical features suggest a genetic thrombophilic disorder:

- Patients with recurrent venous thrombosis or pulmonary embolism.
- Patients with a family history of thrombophilia.

- Patients who present with venous thrombosis under the age of 45 to 50 years.
- Women with a history of multiple miscarriages, stillbirths or both.
- Recurrent venous thrombosis despite adequate anticoagulation.
- Venous thrombosis at unusual sites: cerebral, mesenteric, hepatic (leading to Budd-Chiari syndrome).

Congenital or "genetic" disorders associated with thrombophilia are summarised in the table.

Genetic Disorders Associated with Venous Thrombosis

Condition	Prevalence in population	Prevalence in DVT	Genetics	Comments
Protein C deficiency	1 in 200 to 1 in 500	5%	Autosomal Dominant. Protein C gene mutation on chromosome 2	Protein C and S are vitamin K-dependent glycoproteins with anticoagulant activity. Thrombin binds to thrombomodulin on the endothelium, and protein C is activated by this process. Activated protein C (APC) then binds to its cofactor protein S. The APC/protein S complex then inactivates factor V and VIII in the coagulation cascade. Protein S also functions independently of protein C to inhibit factor X and prothrombin (factor II)
				Homozygous protein C deficiency presents in infancy with purpura fulminans. Heterozygous state presents at a median age of 30 to 40 years with venous thrombosis (lower limb DVT, PE, mesenteric vein thrombosis, cerebral venous thrombosis). Some heterozygous carriers will remain free from venous thrombosis.
				Type 1 protein C deficiency: low protein C level and functional activity.
				Type II protein C deficiency: protein C activity is disproportionately lower than protein C level, due to dysfunctional molecule.
				Warfarin decreases protein C levels and its functional activity. So confirmation of genetic protein C deficiency is difficult in patients already taking warfarin. Skin necrosis can occur with warfarin in patients with protein C deficiency.

Contd...

Contd...

Condition	Prevalence in population	Prevalence in DVT	Genetics	Comments
Protein S deficiency	1 in 700	5%	Autosomal Dominant. Protein S gene mutation on chromosome 3.	Homozygous protein S deficiency presents in infancy with purpura fulminans. Heterozygous state presents at a median age of 30 to 40 years with venous thrombosis; some will remain asymptomatic. Type I protein S deficiency: total protein S and free protein S are low Type II protein S deficiency: normal total and free protein S levels, but low functional activity Type III protein S deficiency: low free protein S, but normal total protein S.
Factor V Leiden (or APC resistance)	2 to 5%	20 to 40%	Factor V gene Mutation at position 506	This is the most common genetic risk factor for an increased risk of venous thrombosis. In the factor V Leiden molecule arginine is replaced by glutamine in position 506. This single amino acid substitution in factor V Leiden affects its binding site for APC, rendering it less susceptible to inactivation by protein C. Hence the term APC resistance. Compared with individuals who do not have the mutation, the homozygous state is associated with a 50 to 100 fold increase in venous thrombosis; and the heterozygous state a 5 to 10 fold increase. The risk of thrombosis with the contraceptive pill is increased by 35 fold, as compared with non-users of the contraceptive pill who do not have the mutation. Minor trauma, pregnancy, surgery and immobilisation will also greatly enhance the risk for venous thrombosis.
Antithrombin III deficiency	1 in 2000 to 1 in 5000	1 to 4%	Autosomal Dominant.	Antithrombin III (AT III) is a natural anticoagulant and inactivates thrombin and factors IX, X, XI, and XII. The anticoagulant effect of AT III is enhanced by heparin. ATIII should not be assayed if the patient is on heparin. Deficiency of AT III leads to recurrent venous thrombosis. The homozygous state is very rare. Heterozygous has AT levels which are 40 to 70% of normal. Type I deficiency: low protein and functional activity. Type II deficiency: normal protein levels, but decreased functional activity. Type III deficiency: mutation in heparin-binding site.

Contd...

Contd...

Condition	Prevalence in population	Prevalence in DVT	Genetics	Comments
Hyperhomo-cysteinaemia	?	?	Mutations in genes encoding homocysteine metabolism	Mutations in the cystathionine α-synthase gene and the methylenetetrahydrofolate reductase (MTHFR) gene are rare and produce very high levels of homocysteine: 100 to 400 µmol/l (normal level < 16).
				Hyperhomocysteinaemia also occurs secondary to: a) deficiencies in folate, vitamin B_{12} and pyridoxine. b) inflammatory bowel disease, uraemia, and phenytoin. Nutritional supplements with folate, vitamin B_{12} and pyridoxine will restore homocysteine levels to normal, but may not abolish completely the thrombotic tendency. Mild (16-24 µmol/l) and moderate (25 to 100 µmol/l) elevations in homocysteine increase the risk of arterial disease (stroke, myocardial infarction, peripheral vascular disease, and carotid artery stenosis) and venous thrombosis.
Prothrombin 20210A	?1 – 2%	?5%	Prothrombin gene mutation	Mutation in the prothrombin gene at position 20210 (G to A substitution) leads to increased activity of plasma prothrombin and a two to three fold increased risk of venous thrombosis in heterozygous people (probably 1 to 2% of the population). The contraceptive pill increases the risk of venous thrombosis in these patients.

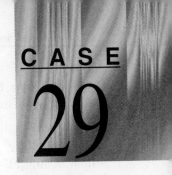
CASE 29

A 67-year-old man was admitted with a 2 weeks history of breathlessness, tiredness, and pain in the thigh muscles of both legs. He had an anterior myocardial infarct 2 years ago. His current medications were aspirin 75 mg od, furosemide 40 mg od, lisinopril 20 mg od, bisoprolol 2.5 mg od, and pravastatin 20 mg od. On examination, his pulse was 70 bpm regular, and BP 105/80 mmHg. There was mild oedema of both ankles. A loud mitral regurgitant murmur was present with a third heart sound. Fine crackles were heard in both lungs. The rest of the examination was unremarkable.

Hb	13.3 g/l
WBC	9.8 x 10⁹/l (normal differential)
Platelets	158 x 10⁹/l
CRP	336 mg/l
Prothrombin time	12.7 seconds
INR	1.2
Na	135 mmol/l
K	3.8 mmol/l
Urea	11.4 mmol/l
Creatinine	209 μmol/l
Glucose	6.8 mmol/l
ALP	79 U/l
AST	55 U/l
CK	1844 U/l
Troponin T	< 0.1 μg/l
Total cholesterol	4.3 mmol/l
HDL cholesterol	1.18 mmol/l
TSH	1.8 mU/l
CXR	cardiomegaly and interstitial oedema

Question
What are the diagnoses?

Answer

Left ventricular failure

Statin induced myositis

Statins, or 3-hydroxy-3-methylglutaryl coenzyme A (HMG-CoA) reductase inhibitors, may rarely produce myositis, which is suggested by muscle pain or weakness with a CK level that is 10 times the upper limit of normal. The estimated incidence of statin induced myositis is around 1-2 per 1,000 patients treated and rhabdomyolysis is seen in about 0.12 patients per million. Cerivastatin was withdrawn in 2002 because of its higher incidence of myositis (2-4 per 1,000 treated) and rhabdomyolysis (3 per million). Statin induced myositis is more frequent when there is accumulation of the drug in renal failure or interference with its metabolism by other medications, such as fibrates, ciclosporin, and nicotinic acid. Statins should be used with caution in patients with liver disease or alcoholism. Abnormal liver function tests occur in about 1% of patients treated. It is recommended that liver function and CK are both measured periodically. Statin therapy should be stopped if the transaminases exceed 3 times the upper limit of normal, or if CK exceeds 10 times the normal limit. Most patients recover fully when the statin medication is withdrawn.

CASE 30

An 81-year-old woman was admitted for investigation of anorexia, watery diarrhoea and 5 kg weight loss over a period of 4 weeks. Past medical history included chronic atrial fibrillation, hypertension, iron deficiency anaemia, and type 2 diabetes. Her medications were bendroflumethiazide 2.5 mg od, metformin 850 mg tds, and ferrous sulphate 200 mg tds. On examination, she was emaciated (BMI = 18) and there was a non-tender distended abdomen. The temperature was 36.4° Celsius, apex heart rate 84 bpm irregular, and BP 155/86 mmHg. Rectal examination showed liquid stool.

Hb	8.1 g/dl
WBC	$9.2 \times 10^9/l$
Platelets	$338 \times 10^9/l$
MCV	72.1 fl
MCH	22.7 pg
CRP	88 mg/l
Na	136 mmol/l
K	3.7 mmol/l
Urea	8.0 mmol/l
Creatinine	101 µmol/l
Blood glucose	8.9 mmol/l
HbA_{1c}	6.5%
Corrected calcium	2.53 mmol/l
Albumin	27 g/l
Bilirubin	6 µmol/l
AST	11 U/l
ALP	111 U/l
TSH	0.01 mU/l
Free T4	29.2 pmol/l
Free T3	3.8 pmol/l
Stool culture	negative

Questions

1. What are the diagnostic possibilities?
2. What further investigations are needed?
3. Comment on the glycated haemoglobin result.

Answers

1. The diagnostic possibilities include:
   - Sick euthyroid syndrome
   - Colonic tumour
   - Metformin induced diarrhoea
   - Coeliac disease
2. The investigations include:
   - Barium enema and colonoscopy
   - Antigliadin, antiendomysial, and anti-tissue transglutaminase antibodies
   - Serum ferritin, folate and vitamin B_{12}
3. The glycated haemoglobin (HbA_{1c}) value is not reliable in any patient with anaemia due to blood loss.

This combination of marked weight loss, iron deficiency anaemia, and recent change in bowel habit suggested the diagnosis of colonic malignancy. Barium enema and colonoscopy showed a malignant stricture in the sigmoid colon, which was removed surgically.

Coeliac disease is common in type 1 diabetes with reported rates of 1.0 – 7.8%. In one series the prevalence of coeliac disease in adults with type 1 diabetes was 1 in 50 (2%) compared with 1 in 340 in type 2 diabetes (0.3%). This suggests there is no increase in coeliac disease among adults with type 2 diabetes.

Coeliac disease can present for the first time in late life. In 1991, 21% of patients who joined Coeliac UK were over the age of 60 years. The presentation of coeliac disease in the elderly often includes anaemia due to either folate or iron deficiency, because both haematinics are mainly absorbed from the jejunum. Some patients with biopsy proven coeliac disease may have negative antibody tests, including anti-tissue transglutaminase. Therefore, if there is a strong clinical suspicion of coeliac disease a jejunal biopsy is recommended.

Metformin is known to cause anorexia, metallic taste, flatulence, and diarrhoea. About 20% of patients on metformin will experience diarrhoea. Vitamin B_{12} deficiency develops in 10-30% of diabetic patients on long term metformin therapy, perhaps after 10-15 years. The uptake of the vitamin B_{12}-intrinsic factor complex by ileal receptors is calcium dependent. Oral calcium supplementation reverses the malabsorption of vitamin B_{12} induced by metformin. The most important side effect of metformin is lactic acidosis, which occurs at a rate of about 3 per 100,000 patients treated and has a mortality rate of 30-50%. Lactic acidosis due to metformin is more likely in patients with liver disease, heart failure and renal failure. Metformin should be avoided if the serum creatinine is above the reference for the patient's age. The following drugs compete with metformin for renal tubular excretion: digoxin, amiloride, morphine, trimethoprim and vancomycin. Metformin should be stopped prior to surgery and is unsafe in conditions associated with hypoxia, hypotension, dehydration, and sepsis. Radiographic contrast nephrotoxicity is an important iatrogenic complication in patients taking metformin. The drug must be stopped for at least 24 hours before the administration of radiographic contrast medium and omitted for another 48 hours after the investigation.

Sick Euthyroid Syndrome

During severe physical illness the following changes in thyroid function are described:

- TSH levels may be low or normal during acute illness
- TSH levels rise during recovery and values could exceed 10 mU/l
- Total T4 is low
- Free T4 can be high, normal, or low (depending on assay methodology)
- Total T3 is low
- Free T3 is low
- Reverse T3 is normal or high

In the Sick Euthyroid Syndrome (SES), a low TSH level may be incorrectly interpreted as hyperthyroidism. *Although the free T4 may be high, normal or low, the free T3 is invariably low in SES.* Another diagnostic possibility for a low TSH, low free T4, and low free T3 is hypopituitarism. In postmenopausal women measurement of FSH and LH is useful as a marker for pituitary function, but this is less helpful in men.

Low levels of FSH and LH in a postmenopausal woman would suggest hypopituitarism.

A sick patient with an elevated TSH, low free T4 and free T3, may have pre-existing hypothyroidism and the presence of thyroid autoantibodies would support this interpretation.

Physiological Mechanisms in SES

• Hypothalamic function is impaired during illness. High plasma cortisol during illness suppresses hypothalamic TRH and impairs TSH release. This leads to low output of thyroid hormones by the thyroid gland. Hence, there is a low T4 and low T3 during acute illness.

• The hepatic enzyme type I 5'-deiodinase (5'-D) converts T4 to T3. The same enzyme removes reverse T3. Therefore, inhibition of 5'-D during illness leads to a fall in T3, rise in T4 (sometimes), and a rise in reverse T3 (sometimes).

• Elevated free fatty acids (FFA >2 mmol/l) displace T4 binding from TBG and lead to a rise in free T4. IV or s/c heparin increases FFA levels *in vitro* and may produce spuriously elevated free T4 levels in some hormone assay methods. Other inhibitors such as metabolites and medications have the same effect.

• Tissue level of T3 is low. Tissue hypothyroidism occurs because (a) entry of T4 into cells is impaired; (b) intracellular conversion of T4 to T3 is abnormal. However, the administration of thyroid hormones to these patients with SES is controversial.

Glycated Haemoglobin (HbA$_1$)

Glycated haemoglobin (HbA$_1$) is produced by the 'adduction' of glucose to the N-terminal valine of the α-chain of adult haemoglobin (HbA$_0$). Glycated haemoglobin (HbA$_1$) is made up of HbA$_{(1a + 1b + 1c)}$. The '1c' sub-fraction of glycated haemoglobin is most stable. As each red cell has a life span of about 3 months, the quantity of glycated haemoglobin is an index of the average blood sugar levels over the same period. Consequently, the glycated haemoglobin is spuriously low in the presence of any medical condition that is associ-

ated with reduced red cell survival, such as:
- Blood loss from the gastrointestinal tract.
- Venesection as in patients with polycythaemia
- Haemolysis

Note: Individuals with haemoglobin S and C will have spuriously low HbA_1 results, whereas haemoglobin F will have spuriously high HbA_{1c} results, with assay techniques that use ionic charge to separate out different haemoglobin subfractions. This is because HbS and HbC coelutes with HbA_0, and HbF coelutes with HbA_1. Glycated haemoglobin results obtained from affinity chromographic methods are not affected by these haemoglobinopathies.

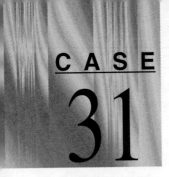

C A S E

31

CASE 31

A 64-year-old man was admitted to the CCU with an acute anterior myocardial infarction. He was a heavy cigarette smoker with COPD and intermittent claudication due to inoperable peripheral vascular disease. There were no immediate complications from thrombolytic therapy using tPA followed by intravenous heparin. However, on the next day he developed atrial fibrillation with a heart rate of 120 bpm, BP 130/60 mmHg, and signs of left ventricular failure. Warfarin, furosemide, lisinopril, and amiodarone were immediately started. A bladder catheter was inserted and average urine volumes were 12 ml per hour. On the third day he was febrile, confused, and the toes of both feet were noticed to be discoloured. The following investigations were obtained:

Urinalysis	protein 2+ and blood 3+
CSU	no growth
Blood culture	no growth
CXR	extensive pulmonary oedema and a right-sided pleural effusion
Hb	10.2 g/dl
WBC	18.7 x 10^9/l
Eosinophil count	1.6 x 10^9/l
Platelets	190 x 10^9/l
CRP	391 mg/l
INR	3.2
Na	134 mmol/l
K	6.1 mmol/l
Urea	36.2 mmol/l
Creatinine	389 μmol/l
CK	301 U/l
Bilirubin	22 μmol/l
ALP	156 U/l
AST	86 U/l
Corrected calcium	2.32 mmol/l

Question

What is the cause of this patient's eosinophilia?

Answer

This patient has cholesterol embolism syndrome (CES). CES describes the occlusion of small and medium sized arteries by cholesterol crystals displaced from ulcerated or ruptured atheromatous plaques in proximal larger arteries. The end result is organ ischaemia with loss of function, or infarction with irreversible damage.

Causes of CES

- Anticoagulation
- Thrombolytic therapy
- Angiography
- Angioplasty, e.g. coronary and renal arteries
- Vascular surgery, e.g. abdominal aneurysm repair, arterial bypass surgery, carotid endarterectomy
- Deceleration injury, e.g. motor vehicle accident

Anticoagulants and thrombolytic agents remove the fibrin-clot sitting in an ulcerated atheromatous plaque and expose the cholesterol-rich extracellular matrix in the subintimal layer of the arterial wall, which is then liberated into the circulation as atheroembolic material. Surgical or radiological vascular procedures can damage the inner arterial wall and displace cholesterol rich atheromatous material into the circulation.

Clinical Presentation of CES

CES can be a difficult diagnosis, because the dysfunction in multiple organs produced by atheroembolism can mimic many other disorders. However, the following clinical triad should raise the possibility of CES:
- Recent anticoagulation or arterial trauma
- Acute renal failure
- Ischaemic skin lesions (see below)

The presentation of CES includes:
- Fever
- Catabolic state
- Cutaneous lesions: livido reticularis (blue-red net-like discoloration), skin infarcts, gangrene, acrocyanosis (purple or blue coloured toes), purpura, petechiae.

- Loin pain, oliguria, haematuria (micro- and macroscopic), hypertension (associated with high renin and angiotensin)
- Heart failure, myocardial infarction
- Confusion, stroke, paraplegia, amaurosis fugax (Hollenhorst plaques are cholesterol emboli in retinal arteries)
- Infarction of bowel, melaena, pancreatitis, splenic infarction
- Myalgia and infarction of lower limb muscles
- Alveolar haemorrhage, haemoptysis, ARDS
- Adrenal infarction and adrenal insufficiency

Fever and a raised CRP (or ESR) are non-specific, and elevations of amylase and liver enzymes depend on involvement of intra-abdominal structures. *Eosinophilia (> 0.4 x 10⁹/l or 4 to18% of the total WBC) is seen in about 80% of patients with CES, but may be transient.* The pedal pulses may be preserved, as the cholesterol micro-emboli tends to affect the much smaller distal vessels. The cutaneous manifestations are common signs in CES (affecting one third of patients) and occur most frequently in the lower limbs. Tissue biopsy (e.g. skin, muscle, or kidney) shows the characteristic biconvex clefts within the arterial lumen left behind by the cholesterol crystals that were removed by the tissue fixation process.

Treatment of CES

- Stop anticoagulation if possible
- Control of hypertension and heart failure
- Haemodialysis with minimal anticoagulation
- Enteral or parenteral nutritional support
- Lipid lowering agent: simvastatin
- Vasodilators: prostacyclin, alprostadil, pentoxifylline (oxpentifylline)
- Sympathectomy

CASE 32

An 81-year-old man with type 2 diabetes was admitted to hospital for treatment of an infected and ischaemic left foot. Past medical history included hypercholesterolaemia, hypertension, and chronic atrial fibrillation. His medications were metformin 850 mg bd, pravastatin 20 mg od, lisinopril 20 mg od, digoxin 62.5 µg od, and furosemide 40 mg od. On the second day angiography was performed using a left femoral approach and showed severe arterial occlusion in both legs. His blood tests are tabulated below:

	On admission	Day 3	Day 6
Na	133 mmol/l	132 mmol/l	126 mmol/l
K	4.9 mmol/l	6.0 mmol/l	7.5 mmol/l
Urea	5.8 mmol/l	19.3 mmol/l	35.2 mmol/l
Creatinine	100 µmol/l	159 µmol/l	411 µmol/l
HbA$_{1c}$	7.1%		
Hb	12.8 g/dl		
WBC	9 x 10^9/l		
Platelets	331 x 10^9/l		
CRP	51 mg/l		
LFT	normal		
Total cholesterol	2.5 mmol/l		

Question

What is the most likely cause for this man's deteriorating renal function?

Answer

This patient has metformin related radiocontrast nephrotoxicity.

Iodinated radiographic contrast media produce renal vaso-constriction and liberate reactive oxygen species, or "free radicals", which are toxic to renal tubular cells. The following are important risk factors for radiocontrast nephrotoxicity:

- Pre-existing renal impairment and proteinuria
- Diabetes mellitus
- Hypertension
- Heart failure
- Elderly patients
- Multiple myeloma
- Large contrast load
- Nephrotoxic medications: metformin, ACE-I, NSAID, aminoglycosides, amphotericin, ciclosporin, tacrolimus, cisplatin, methotrexate, foscarnet, sulphonamides, acyclovir, indinavir.

Preventing Radiocontrast Nephrotoxicity

- Stop any nephrotoxic drug before the radiographic investigation. Metformin should be stopped for at least 24 hours before any radiographic contrast study and omitted for another 48 hours afterwards.
- Discontinue any diuretics beforehand. Furosemide potentiates the renal toxicity of radiocontrast media and the ototoxicity of aminoglycosides.
- Non-ionic contrast media may be safer in patients with diabetes or pre-existing renal impairment.
- Hydration. Infusion of half normal saline (0.45% NaCl) before, during and after the radiographic contrast study. Typically at a rate of 50 – 100 ml per hour starting 12 hours before and continuing for at least 12 hours after the administration of radiographic contrast.
- N-acetylcysteine has been shown to prevent radiocontrast nephrotoxicity in a group of patients with chronic renal impairment (mean creatinine 216 µmol/l), perhaps by its antioxidant action. It is given in a dose of 600 mg bd orally the day before and on the day of radiocontrast exposure.

CASE 33

A 45-year-old man was admitted for investigation of fever. About 4 weeks ago he had fallen accidentally onto his face and since then has had pain over the left orbit and cheek. Past medical history included sinus infections. On examination, his temperature was 38° Celsius, pulse 86 bpm, and BP 138/64 mmHg. There was tenderness over the maxillary sinuses, but no signs of meningism were present. The rest of the physical examination was unremarkable.

Hb	$10.1 \times 10^9/l$
WBC	$4.2 \times 10^9/l$
Platelets	$458 \times 10^9/l$
ESR	72 mm/h
Na	138 mmol/l
K	4.1 mmol/l
Urea	4.2 mmol/l
Creatinine	92 μmol/l
Albumin	32 g/l
Globulin	32 g/l
ALP	95 U/l
ALT	22 U/l
Corrected calcium	2.51 mmol/l
Protein electrophoresis	raised alpha $_1$ and alpha$_2$ globulin
ANA	< 1 in 40
ANCA	positive cytoplasmic pattern (C-ANCA)
MPO (P-ANCA) antibodies	6 U/l (ref 0 – 6)
PR3 (C- ANCA) antibodies	59 U/l (ref 0 - 6)
CXR	patchy shadow right upper lobe
Skull X-ray	chronic polypoidal sinus disease, no evidence of orbital fracture

Question
What is the diagnosis?

Answer

The diagnosis is **Wegener's** granulomatosis. Wegener's granulomatosis is a vasculitis of the medium and small arteries. The clinical diagnosis is suggested by the presence of at least 2 of the 4 following criteria:
- **Nasal or oral inflammation** (nasal obstruction, purulent or bloody nasal discharge, saddle nose from damaged nasal septum, sinus pain, oral ulcers)
- **Pulmonary infiltrates**, nodules or cavities (haemoptysis and breathlessness)
- **Haematuria** (crescentic necrotizing glomerulonephritis presenting as microscopic haematuria or proteinuria)
- **Granulomatous inflammation** without infection on biopsy

Other clinical manifestations are:
- **Ocular** (proptosis)
- **Middle ear involvement** (deafness)
- **Tracheal (hoarseness and stridor)**
- **Neurological** (mononeuritis multiplex and cranial neuropathy)
- **Cutaneous** (palpable purpura)
- **Arthritis or arthralgia** (monoarticular or polyarticular)

Histological confirmation of granulomatous vasculitis requires biopsy material taken from a site of active disease such as the nasopharynx, lung, or kidney.

Antineutrophilic Cytoplasmic Antibodies (ANCA)

These are antibodies directed against cytoplasmic antigens within neutrophils. Two types of antibodies are recognised:
- **C-ANCA** stains the cytoplasm and is directed against the antigen serine proteinase, PR3.
- **P-ANCA** stains the perinuclear region and is directed against myeloperoxidase.

Most patients with Wegener's granulomatosis will be C-ANCA (PR3) positive.

Treatment of Wegener's Granulomatosis

Disease remission is induced with prednisolone and cyclophosphamide.

- IV or oral prednisolone at an initial dose of 1 mg/kg/day and then tail down gradually.
- IV or oral cyclophosphamide at an initial dose of 2 mg/kg/day. Alternatives are azathioprine and methotrexate.
- Pneumocystis carinii pneumonia is a serious complication of immunosuppression. Prophylaxis with trimethoprim/sulfamethoxazole (160/800 mg, three times a week) is recommended.
- Renal supportive treatment, including transplantation.

Prognosis of Wegener's Granulomatosis

The mortality at 5 years is around 25-30%. Death is from either the complications of the disease (e.g. renal failure) or the complications from the treatment (e.g. infection or malignancy).

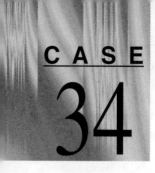

CASE 34

A previously healthy 22-year-old man was admitted to hospital with a high fever, sore throat, headache, neck pain, and intermittent confusion. Ten days earlier his General Practitioner had diagnosed tonsillitis and started a course of amoxicillin, which was stopped after 2 days because of an itchy rash. On examination, the temperature was 38.2° Celsius, pulse 120 bpm regular, BP 106/64 mmHg, both tonsils were enlarged and inflamed, and there was a large tender swelling at the angle of the right jaw and neck. A faint rash was present all over the trunk and limbs. The chest, heart and abdomen were unremarkable.

Hb	12.7 g/dl
WBC	22.3 x 10⁹/l (75% neutrophils)
Platelets	301 x 10⁹/l
CRP	359 mg/l
Na	140 mmol/l
K	4.1 mmol/l
Urea	8 mmol/l
Creatinine	87 µmol/l
Bilirubin	43 µmol/l
ALT	87 U/l
ALP	159 U/l
Urinalysis	blood + and protein +
CXR	normal
CT brain scan	normal
CSF	normal

Questions
1. What are the diagnostic possibilities?
2. What investigations would you perform?

Answers

1. The diagnostic possibilities are:
   - Peritonsillar abscess (Quinsy)
   - Glandular fever
   - Lemierre's syndrome
2. Investigations would include:
   - Blood film for atypical lymphocytes
   - Monospot test
   - Culture of throat swab
   - Blood culture
   - Epstein-Barr virus serology
   - CT or MRI of the neck

Lemierre's syndrome is usually due to infection of the oropharynx or mastoid by Fusobacterium necrophorum, a gram negative anaerobic bacillus that leads to septic thrombophlebitis of the internal jugular vein. In this condition septic thrombus breaks off from the internal jugular vein to produce metastatic abscesses in the lungs, liver, kidney, joints and spine. Multiple subcutaneous abscesses, meningitis, and empyema also arise from haematogenous spread. CT and MRI scans are the best methods for identifying internal jugular vein thrombophlebitis. Fusobacterium necrophorum is usually sensitive to penicillin (although some isolates produce β-lactamase), quinolones, clindamycin, and metronidazole. A prolonged 3 to 6 weeks course of antibiotic treatment is recommended. Ligation of the internal jugular vein is reserved for patients with recurrent pulmonary emboli. Surgical drainage of metastatic abscesses may be necessary. The role of anticoagulation is uncertain.

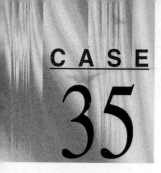

CASE

35

CASE 35

Over a 24 hour period a previously healthy 49-year-old developed a high fever and widespread petechial rash. His General Practitioner administered IV benzylpenicillin and arranged an urgent hospital admission. On arrival the patient was confused, febrile (38.6° Celsius), hypotensive (BP 80/70 mmHg) and tachycardic (120 bpm regular). There was a widespread non-blanching petechial rash. No signs of meningism were present. Chest and heart sounds were normal. The liver and spleen were slightly enlarged.

Hb	9.2 g/dl
MCV	101 fl
WBC	1.7 x 10⁹/l
Platelets	12 x 10⁹/l
Reticulocyte	1.3%
CRP	13 mg/l
Prothrombin time	14 seconds
APTT	35 seconds
Na	132 mmol/l
K	3.8 mmol/l
Urea	9 mmol/l
Creatinine	127 µmol/l
Bilirubin	37 µmol/l
ALT	324 U/l
ALP	453 U/l
Amylase	84 U/l
Albumin	28 g/l
Globulin	42 g/l
Corrected calcium	2.3 mmol/l
Urinalysis	normal
CXR	normal
ECG	sinus tachycardia

Questions
1. What are the diagnostic possibilities?
2. What further investigations are needed?

Answers

1. Pancytopenia has many possible causes, including:
   - Severe septicaemia: meningococcal
   - Viral infection: viral hepatitis, Epstein-Barr virus, Parvovirus B-19
   - Megaloblastic anaemia
   - Systemic lupus erythematosus
   - Drug induced bone marrow failure
   - Marrow infiltration: leukaemia, lymphoma, myeloma
   - Hypersplenism
   - Paroxysmal nocturnal haemoglobinuria
   - Thymoma

2. The essential investigations are:
   - Blood culture
   - Meningococcal antigen
   - Viral serology
   - Vitamin B_{12} and folate
   - Haptoglobins
   - Coombs' test
   - Anti-DNA antibody
   - ANCA
   - Protein electrophoresis
   - Bone marrow examination
   - Ham's test
   - Ultrasound or CT chest and abdomen

Haemophagocytosis Syndrome

This previously healthy patient has a pancytopenia and hepatosplenomegaly. The bone marrow showed large numbers of activated macrophages that were ingesting erythrocytes, platelets and leucocytes, a phenomenon called haemophagocytosis.

T-cell stimulation by a variety of stimuli leads to the production of excessive cytokines (interferon-γ, TNF-α, interleukin-1β), which in turn activate macrophages in the bone marrow, lymph nodes, liver and spleen. Tissue damage by activated macrophages involves the lung, heart, liver, spleen, kidney, and nervous system. Within the bone marrow, spleen and lymph nodes, the ingestion of blood precursors by activated macrophages account for the profound pancytopenia.

Types of Haemophagocytosis Syndrome (HS)

Primary haemophagocytic syndrome
- Familial disorder (autosomal recessive inheritance). This condition appears in infancy.

Secondary haemophagocytic syndrome
- Virus associated HS (Epstein-Barr, cytomegalovirus, herpes simplex, adenovirus)
- Non-viral infection associated HS (bacteria, fungal).
- Malignancy associated HS (leukaemia, lymphoma, myeloma)

Treatment of HS

- Supportive measures, including antibiotics and antiviral medication
- Immunosuppression (corticosteroids, ciclosporin). Ciclosporin may suppress the T-cell activation and cytokine production seen in HS.

C A S E

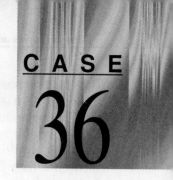

36

CASE 36

A 56-year-old man was started on amiodarone 6 months ago which completely abolished his attacks of paroxsymal atrial fibrillation. Comment on the following thyroid function tests taken at a recent clinic visit:

TSH	0.01 mU/l
Free T4	> 80 pmol/l
Free T3	> 39 pmol/l

Question
What is the diagnosis?

-111-

Answer

This patient has amiodarone induced thyrotoxicosis (AIT).
Amiodarone has the following pharmacological properties:
- 37% of the amiodarone molecule is iodine and each day 10% of the amiodarone is deiodinated.
- A 200 mg dose of amiodarone contains 74 mg of iodine, from which 7.4 mg of iodine is made available.
- Dealkylation produces the main metabolite desethylamiodarone (DEA).
- 70% of the drug is removed by biliary excretion.
- The half life of amiodarone is 40 days and 57 days for DEA.

Effects of Amiodarone on Thyroid Function

- Amiodarone inhibits hepatic Type I 5'-deiodinase (Type I 5'-D), which converts T4 to T3. As a consequence T4 rises and T3 falls. Reverse T3 also rises as it is not removed by type I 5'-D
- High dose amiodarone inhibits Type II 5'-D, which converts T4 to T3 within the pituitary gland. This leads to a rise in TSH during the first few months.
- Amiodarone and its principal metabolite desethylamiodarone (DEA) inhibit the entry of thyroid hormone into cells, to produce a state of tissue hypothyroidism.
- Amiodarone and DEA are both toxic to thyroid cells, causing preformed thyroid hormone to be released into the circulation.

Amiodarone Induced Thyrotoxicosis (AIT)

Type 1 AIT

- Associated with pre-existing thyroid disease (e.g. diffuse or nodular goitre, and latent Graves' disease).
- Radioiodine uptake is normal or high in iodine deficient areas.
  Radioiodine uptake is low in iodine sufficient areas.
- Serum interleukin-6 (IL-6) levels are normal or slightly elevated.
- Jod Basedow phenomenon is likely: excess iodine leading to excessive thyroid hormone synthesis.
- Hyperactive vascular gland is shown by Colour Flow Doppler.

- Treatment is difficult and the options include:
  - Stop amiodarone if possible
  - High dose carbimazole 60 mg od
  - Potassium perchlorate 1 g od for 6 weeks, but this can produce aplastic anaemia.
  - Lithium carbonate reduces thyroid hormone release (900 mg od for 6 weeks).
  - Plasmapheresis to remove excess thyroid hormones.
  - Radioiodine if the uptake is adequate.
  - Thyroidectomy, but these patients are often a poor anaesthetic risk.

Type 2 AIT

- Radioiodine uptake is very low (< 2-3%)
- IL-6 levels are very high, suggesting thyroid gland destruction.
- Thyrotoxicosis is due to the destruction of a normal thyroid gland with the release of preformed thyroid hormones. Thyrotoxicosis is sometimes followed by hypothyroidism.
- Absence of hypervascularity on Colour Flow Doppler.
- Treatment includes:
  - steroids in high dose; relapse may occur if steroids are withdrawn too quickly.
  - carbimazole
  - plasmapheresis to remove thyroid hormone

N.B. Mixed forms occur, which require a combination of carbimazole, potassium perchlorate, and steroids.

Amiodarone Induced Hypothyroidism

- Occurs most often in iodine sufficient areas.
- Pre-existing autoimmune thyroiditis in some patients.
- Iodination of thyroglobulin is inhibited by the large doses of iodine provided by amiodarone therapy. This phenomenon is called the Wolff-Chaikoff effect.
- Stop amiodarone if possible – hypothyroidism may remit in patients without autoimmune disease (i.e. thyroid autoantibody negative)
- Treat with thyroxine and maintain TSH in upper half of the normal range.

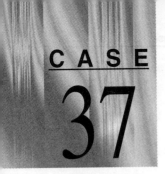

C A S E
37

CASE 37

A 52-year-old woman with type 1 diabetes had pins and needles in both hands, which were worse at night. Her nerve conduction tests are shown below.

Sensory Conduction Study

	Latency (ms = millisecond) (normal <3.7 ms)	Amplitude (μV = microvolt) (normal > 8-10 μV)
R. median nerve SAP (index finger to wrist)	4.6 ms	3.8 μV
R. ulnar nerve SAP (little finger to wrist)	2.5 ms	4.5 μV
L. median nerve SAP (index finger to wrist)	6.5 ms	5.8 μV
L. ulnar nerve SAP (little finger to wrist)	2.1 ms	4.4 μV
(SAP = sensory action potential)		

Motor Conduction Study

	Latency (ms = millisecond) (normal < 4.0 ms)	Amplitude (mV = millivolt) (normal > 5mV)
Distal motor latency:		
R. median nerve (wrist to thenar)	6.7 ms	7.0 mV
R. median nerve (elbow to wrist)	5.2 ms	5.8 mV
R. ulnar nerve (wrist to hypothenar)	2.3 ms	4.1 mV
R. ulnar nerve (elbow to wrist)	4.2 ms	2.7 mV
L. median nerve (wrist to thenar)	6.1 ms	3.9 mV
L. median nerve (elbow to wrist)	4.5 ms	3.8 mV
L. ulnar nerve (wrist to hypothenar)	0.8 ms	6.5 mV
L. ulnar nerve (elbow to wrist)	4.3 ms	5.8 mV

Conduction velocity:

R. median nerve motor conduction velocity = 40.4 metre/s
R. ulnar nerve motor conduction velocity = 53.7 metre/s
L. median nerve motor conduction velocity = 46.5 metre/s
L. ulnar nerve motor conduction velocity = 53.0 metre/s

Questions
1. What are the abnormalities in this nerve conduction study?
2. How would you interpret these findings?

Answers

1. The abnormalities are:
 - Depression in the sensory action potential (SAP) in both median and ulnar nerves.
 - Prolongation of the distal motor latency in both median nerves across the wrists.
 - Prolonged sensory latency in both median nerves across the wrists.
 - Depression of the motor conduction velocities in both median nerves.

2. Interpretations
 - The depression in SAP in both median and ulnar nerves is compatible with diabetic sensory peripheral neuropathy.
 - The prolongation of the distal motor latency in both median nerves across the wrist suggests bilateral carpal tunnel syndrome (CTS). Normal values for electrophysiological tests depend on the laboratory. However, a distal motor latency > 4.0 millisecond is generally regarded as being abnormal. The median nerve motor conduction velocity in established CTS is usually < 50 metres per second.
 - The earliest and most sensitive indicator of CTS is a prolonged distal sensory latency. A distal sensory latency > 3.7 millisecond is abnormal and > 6 millisecond suggests severe CTS.
 - The diagnostic accuracy of nerve conduction studies for CTS may be improved when Phalen's test is performed (see below).

Carpal Tunnel Syndrome

The carpal tunnel is formed by the bones of the wrist and the transverse carpal ligament. The median nerve and nine flexor tendons pass through this tunnel. Entrapment of the median nerve at the wrist is called carpal tunnel syndrome. The mechanisms include fluid retention, swelling of the tendons, and deformity of the carpal bones, such as in:
 - Rheumatoid arthritis
 - Previous wrist fractures
 - Multiple myeloma
 - Pregnancy

- Diabetes
- Hypothyroidism

Clinical Manifestations of CTS

The symptoms are pain, paraesthesia and muscle weakness. The pain and paraesthesia usually occur in the cutaneous distribution of the median nerve: thumb, index and middle fingers and the radial half of the ring finger. In some patients the whole hand is painful. Occasionally, the pain radiates proximally to the elbow, upper arm and shoulder. Symptoms are worse at night, and relief is produced by hanging the hand over the bed. The signs include:

- The "flick sign" describes the relief of symptoms by shaking the hand.
- Tinel's test refers to the pain and paraesthesia induced by tapping the median nerve at the wrist.
- Phalen's test describes the pain and paraesthesia produced by active full flexion of the wrist for 60 seconds, or the induction of identical symptoms by inflating a sphygmomanometer cuff above systolic blood pressure for 60 seconds.
- Weakness and wasting of the abductor pollicis brevis is tested by placing the back of the hand on a flat surface and pushing the thumb straight upwards against resistance.
- Weakness of the opponens pollicis is tested by asking the patient to pinch the tips of the thumb and little finger together, and then the examiner attempts to separate them.

Treatment of CTS

- Conservative measures:
  - Avoid use of the wrist.
  - Wrist splints.
  - NSAID.
  - Steroid injection (e.g. prednisolone 25 mg in 1 ml with bupivacaine 0.5% in 0.5 ml) in the carpal tunnel.

  The following groups respond poorly to conservative measures:
  - Patients over the age of 50 years.
  - Severe symptoms for more than 10 months.

- Presence of thenar muscle wasting.
- Abnormal nerve conduction study.
• Endoscopic carpal tunnel release
• Division of the transverse carpal ligament

CASE 38

A 78-year-old woman was admitted to hospital for investigation of watery diarrhoea and weight loss of 5 kg during the last 6 months. In the last one month she developed peripheral oedema and breathlessness on minimal effort. On examination, she looked pale with puffy eyelids and glossitis. The temperature was 36.3° Celsius, pulse 90 bpm regular, and BP 126/84 mmHg. There were signs of bilateral pleural effusions, oedema of both legs up to the groins, and a swollen abdomen containing an ascites. Flexible sigmoidoscopy showed no mucosal abnormalities. Endoscopic examination demonstrated normal findings in the upper gastrointestinal tract. The endoscopic duodenal biopsy showed subtotal villus atrophy. There was no response to a gluten free diet, corticosteroids, and nutritional supplements.

Hb	9.4 g/dl
WBC	7.6 x 10^9/l (normal differential)
Platelets	247 x 10^9/l
MCV	87 fl
CRP	< 8 mg/l
Serum folate	9.4 nmol/l
Vitamin B$_{12}$	105 pmol/l
Ferritin	64 µg/l
Na	133 mmol/l
K	4.7 mmol/l
Urea	3.9 mmol/l
Creatinine	73 µmol/l
Bilirubin	17 µmol/l
Albumin	18 g/l
Globulin	26 g/l
ALT	37 U/l
ALP	143 U/l

Corrected calcium	2.3 mmol/l
TSH	0.44 mU/l
Urinalysis	normal
ECG	normal
CXR	bilateral pleural effusions
ECHO	good left ventricular function and a small pericardial effusion
US scan abdomen	ascites, normal liver, spleen and kidneys
Stool culture	negative
Autoantibodies	antigliadin, antiendomysial, gastric parietal, intrinsic factor – all negative

Question

What is the most likely diagnosis?

Answer

The diagnosis is lymphoma of the small bowel with protein losing enteropathy.

Increased protein loss across the bowel mucosa, which exceeds the hepatic synthesis of albumin, produces hypoalbuminaemia. The most common presenting complaint is peripheral oedema, because hypoalbuminaemia is associated with the loss of plasma oncotic pressure and the transudation of fluid into the subcutaneous tissues. The causes of protein losing enteropathy include:

Mucosal Damage

- Inflammatory bowel disease
- Carcinoma of stomach
- Pseudomembranous colitis
- Coeliac disease
- Bacterial overgrowth
- Giant hypertrophic gastritis (Menetrier's disease)
- Whipple's disease (Tropheryma whippeii)
- Amyloidosis
- Graft versus host disease

Lymphatic Obstruction

- Congestive cardiac failure
- Constrictive pericarditis
- Lymphoma
- Tuberculosis
- Sarcoidosis
- Retroperitoneal fibrosis
- Lymphangiectasia, which is demonstrated by lymphangiography.

Loss of protein through the gut can be demonstrated by:
- IV radiolabelled serum albumin, which is lost in the stool if there is protein losing enteropathy.
- Stool alpha $_1$- antitrypsin is neither secreted nor absorbed by normal bowel, and its appearance in the stool suggests the diagnosis of protein losing enteropathy.

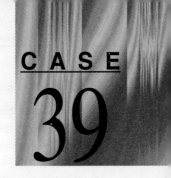

CASE 39

These are the lung function tests of a 46-year-old woman who has symptoms of breathlessness.

SPIROMETRY

	Predicted Value	Pre-Salbutamol	% Predicted	Post-Salbutamol	% Predicted	Percent Change
FVC L	3.14	3.28	104	3.7	117	12
FEV1 L	2.69	1.6	59	2.34	86	46
FEV1/FVC %	80	49	61	63	78	28

DIFFUSION

	Predicted Value	Actual Value	% Predicted
DLCO	8.35	7.51	89
VA	4.23	4.68	110
KCO	1.68	1.6	95

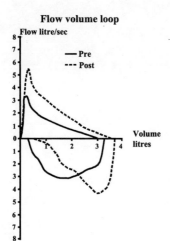

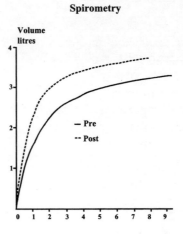

Question
What is the diagnosis?

Answer

The diagnosis is bronchial asthma.

An increase in FEV1 (or PEFR) by $\geq$ 15% after bronchodilator medication or trial of oral prednisolone (typically 30 mg a day for 14 days) is regarded as a significant increase and would suggest a diagnosis of reversible airflow obstruction i.e. asthma. However, the absolute increase in FEV1 must be at least 0.2 litres (or 60 litres in PEFR). In chronic obstructive pulmonary disease (COPD) the airflow obstruction is relatively fixed and there is no significant increase in spirometric values with salbutamol or prednisolone.

In this patient the FEV1/FVC before salbutamol was 49% compared with a predicted value of 80%. This reduction in FEV1/FVC is typical of airflow obstruction. After salbutamol there is a 46% increase in FEV1 (and 12% in FVC). This dramatic improvement in airflow obstruction with inhaled salbutamol is diagnostic of asthma.

CASE 40

This 64-year-old man has smoked cigarettes all his adult life and now complains of breathlessness. These are his lung function tests.

SPIROMETRY

	Predicted Value	Pre-Salbutamol	% Predicted	Post-Salbutamol	% Predicted	Percent Change
FVC L	3.56	1.98	55	2.38	66	20
FEV1 L	2.8	0.7	25	0.69	24	-1
FEV1/FVC %	76	35	46	29	38	-17

LUNG VOLUMES

	Predicted Value	Pre-Salbutamol	% Predicted
SVC L	3.56	1.91	53
RV L	2.35	5.61	238
TLC L	6.19	7.52	121
RV/TLC %	39	75	192

DIFFUSION

	Predicted Value	Actual Value	% Predicted
DLCO	24.53	10.12	41
VA	5.26	4.1	77
KCO	3.96	2.47	62

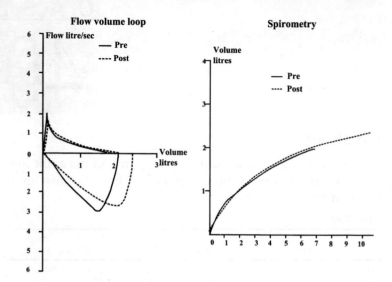

Question

What is the diagnosis?

Answer

This man has severe airflow obstruction as shown by a FEV1/ FVC of 35%. After salbutamol his FEV1 fell a little bit, but the FVC increased by 20%. In some patients with COPD this increase in FVC may be associated with improvement in symptoms and effort tolerance. The total lung capacity is high and the residual volume is greatly increased, indicating air trapping and hyperinflation. The gas transfer factor (DLCO) and the alveolar volume (VA) are both decreased. The KCO is the gas transfer factor (DLCO) divided by alveolar volume (VA). A low KCO suggests emphysema.

In the British Thoracic Society COPD guidelines (1997), the severity of airflow obstruction is graded as follows:

Mild:	FEV1	60-80% of predicted
Moderate:	FEV1	40-59% of predicted
Severe:	FEV1	< 40% of predicted

N.B. The "normal" FEV1 is $\geq$ 80% of predicted.

Upper Airway Obstruction

Upper airway obstruction refers to narrowing of the larger central airways (i.e. larynx, trachea, right and left main bronchi) and can be demonstrated by changes in flow volume curves.

Types of Upper Airway Obstruction

- Variable extrathoracic: vocal cord palsy, goitre, airway burns, tracheomalacia, neoplasm
- Variable intrathoracic: tracheomalacia, neoplasm
- Fixed extrathoracic ⎫ tracheal stenosis, foreign body,
- Fixed intrathoracic ⎭ neoplasm

Large airways inside the chest dilate during inspiration while airways outside the chest tend to collapse due to the fall in intraluminal pressure. During expiration the reverse is true: airways inside the chest collapse while airways outside the chest are held open by the expiratory flow. Consequently:

- Variable extrathoracic obstruction blunts the inspiratory part of the flow volume curve.

- Variable intrathoracic obstruction blunts the expiratory part of the flow volume curve.
- Fixed intrathoracic or fixed extrathoracic obstruction affects both inspiratory and expiratory parts of the flow volume curve (see example below).

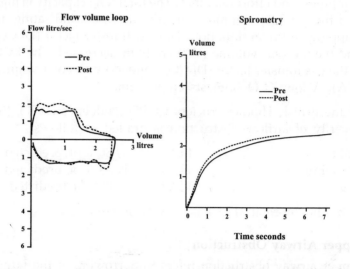

CASE 41

This 72-year-old woman presented with breathlessness. These are her lung function tests.

SPIROMETRY

	Predicted Value	Pre-Salbutamol	% Predicted	Post-Salbutamol	% Predicted	Percent Change
FVC L	1.88	0.74	39	0.76	40	2
FEV1 L	1.52	0.65	42	0.67	44	3
FEV1/FVC %	75	88	117	89	118	1

LUNG VOLUMES

	Predicted Value	Pre-Salbutamol	% Predicted
SVC L	1.88	0.75	39
RV L	1.86	0.94	50
TLC L	4.1	1.68	40
RV/TLC %	43	56	130

DIFFUSION

	Predicted Value	Actual Value	% Predicted
DLCO	17.91	8.59	47
VA	3.49	1.37	39
KCO	4.37	6.27	143

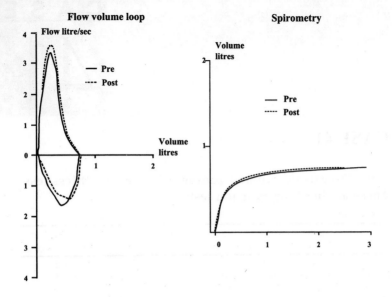

Question
What are the abnormalities?

Answer

The low VC and TLC suggest small lungs and are typical features of a restrictive defect.

Causes of restrictive pulmonary defects include:

- pulmonary fibrosis
- heart failure
- pleural effusions
- skeletal abnormality: kyphosis

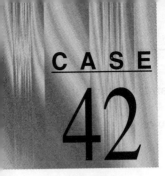

C A S E

42

CASE 42

A 78-year-old woman was referred to hospital for investigation of acute visual deterioration, dizziness and headache. Past medical history included insulin treated type 2 diabetes, hypertension, mastectomy for carcinoma of the left breast 42 years ago, and hysterectomy for carcinoma of the uterus 7 years ago. Her medications were atenolol 100 mg od, lisinopril 10 mg od, doxazosin 4 mg od, furosemide 20 mg od, and human insulatard insulin. On examination, her pulse was 76 bpm regular, BP 180/90 mmHg, and temperature 37° Celsius. The liver and spleen were both enlarged and easily palpable at 3 cm below the costal margins. There was a left homonymous hemianopia and mild background diabetic retinopathy.

Hb	17.9 x 10⁹/l
WBC	13.7 x 10⁹/l
Neutrophils	10.14 x 10⁹/l (ref 2 – 7.5)
Lymphocytes	2.6 x 10⁹/l (ref 1 – 4)
Monocytes	0.96 x 10⁹/l (0.2 – 0.8)
Eosinophils	0 x 10⁹/l
Basophils	0 x 10⁹/l
Platelets	223 x 10⁹/l
Haematocrit	55%
MCV	70.4 fl
CRP	< 8 mg/l
Na	137 mmol/l
K	4.6 mmol/l
Urea	11.2 mmol/l
Creatinine	138 µmol/l
Albumin	40 g/l
Globulin	31 g/l
ALP	160 U/l
ALT	19 U/l

Corrected calcium	2.42 mmol/l
Plasma glucose	20.4 mmol/l
HbA$_{1c}$	11.8%
CXR	slightly enlarged heart
ECG	sinus rhythm and voltage criteria for left ventricular hypertrophy

Questions

1. What is the diagnosis?
2. What further investigations are required?

Answers

1. Polycythaemia vera
2. CT brain scan showed an infarct in the right occipital lobe.

Bone marrow showed a hypercellular aspirate, with markedly increased numbers of cells in the megakaryocytic, myeloid, and erythroid series.

The abdominal ultrasound confirmed the presence of hepatosplenomegaly.

Leucocyte alkaline phosphatase was high.

Polycythaemia Vera

The myeloproliferative disorders include polycythaemia vera, chronic myeloid leukaemia, essential thrombocythaemia, and myelofibrosis. These 4 conditions are characterised by a genetic alteration that conveys a growth advantage to a single clone of pluripotent haematopoietic stem cells. In primary polycythaemia (or polycythaemia vera, PV) there is excessive and unregulated proliferation of the erythroid, myeloid and megakaryocytic progenitor cells. Erythroid progenitor cells in PV are hyper-responsive to growth factors including erythropoietin (EPO), insulin-like growth factor, and interleukin-3.

Secondary polycythaemia is due to excessive EPO production in response to tissue hypoxia (as in chronic lung disease and cyanotic heart disease), or an EPO secreting tumour (as in renal tumour, adrenal tumour, hepatoma, large uterine fibroids, and cerebellar haemangioblastoma). Relative or "stress" polycythaemia describes the haemoconcentration due to a relative decrease in plasma volume, e.g. dehydration, and burns.

Clinical Manifestations of PV

- The median age of onset is 60 years
- Male to female ratio is about 1:2.
- Ruddy facial complexion
- Generalised pruritis after a hot bath

- Erythromelalgia: erythema, pain and increased temperature, usually in the lower limbs.
- Gout due to increased cellular turnover
- Thrombotic problems: stroke, Budd-Chiari syndrome, splenic infarction
- Haemorrhagic problems: gastrointestinal bleeding from peptic ulcers
- Hypertension
- Hepatosplenomegaly. The spleen is enlarged in 70% of patients and liver is enlarged in 50%.
- Hyperviscosity syndrome (headache, visual disturbance, tinnitus, vertigo)

Laboratory Findings in PV

- Elevated Hb, WBC and platelet count. The WBC is elevated in 70% of patients, often with increased numbers of basophils or monocytes. The platelet count is high in 50% of patients and may include abnormally large platelets with defective function.
- Raised serum uric acid
- Low iron stores. In the presence of iron deficiency the Hb and red cell mass may lie in the normal range, although the WBC and platelets will remain high and can be misdiagnosed as chronic myeloid leukaemia or essential thrombocythaemia. *However, the leucocyte alkaline phosphatase is high in PV and low in chronic myeloid leukaemia.* When PV progresses to myelofibrosis with bone marrow failure, pancytopenia appears.
- EPO levels are normal or low
- 20-40% of patients show cytogenetic abnormalities including chromosomal trisomy and deletions.

Diagnostic Criteria of the PV Study Group

Category A

- A1. Elevated red cell mass: ≥ 36 ml/kg in men; ≥ 32ml/kg in women
- A2. Normal arterial oxygen saturation: ≥ 92%

- A3. Palpable splenomegaly
- A4. Cytogenetic abnormality

Category B

- B1. Thrombocytosis: platelets $\geq 400 \times 10^9/l$
- B2. Leucocytosis: WBC $\geq 12.0 \times 10^9/l$ in absence of fever or infection
- B3. Splenomegaly shown on ultrasound
- B4. Reduced EPO level

The diagnosis of PV is accepted for the following combinations:
A1 + A2 + A3 or A4
A1 + A2 + any two items from category B.

Treatment of PV

- Venesection. Aim for a haematocrit of below 45%, but venesection does not control the thrombocytosis or leucocytosis. N.B. In this diabetic patient with polycythaemia vera, venesection would shorten the life span of red blood cells and lower the glycated haemoglobin (HbA$_{1c}$) values.
- Hydroxycarbamide (hydroxyurea) for reducing thrombocytosis.
- Alpha interferon (IFN-α) is expensive and associated with flu-like side effects. IFN-α is suited for women of child-bearing age as it is devoid of leukaemic risk and teratogenicity.
- Radioactive phosphorus (^{32}P) is reserved for older patients (> 70 years). It is not recommended for younger patients as it has a leukaemogenic risk.
- Allopurinol to prevent gout.

Prognosis of PV

- The median survival is about 10 years: 5-10% of patients will develop acute myeloblastic leukaemia and a similar number develop myelofibrosis.

CASE 43

A 31-year-old woman complained of tiredness. These are her blood test results:

Hb	4.4 x 10^9/l
WBC	20.5 x 10^9/l (neutrophilia and right shifted cells)
Platelets	114 x 10^9/l
MCV	140.4 fl
Vitamin B$_{12}$	933 pmol/l (ref 130- 660)
Serum folate	1.6 nmol/l (ref 4.8 – 40)
Red cell folate	412 nmol/l (ref 770 – 1800)
Ferritin	747 µg/l (ref 20 – 300)
CRP	27 mg/l
Na	132 mmol/l
K	2.7 mmol/l
Urea	2.6 mmol/l
Creatinine	75 µmol/l
Albumin	31 g/l
Globulin	35 g/l
Bilirubin	36 µmol/l
Conjugated bilirubin	18 µmol/l (normal < 3.4)
Haptoglobins	0.53 g/l (ref 0.5 – 2.0)
ALT	38 U/l
ALP	154 U/l
γ-GT	194 U/l
TSH	11.95 mU/l
Free T4	17.7 pmol/l
Corrected calcium	2.47 mmol/l
Glucose	5.2 mmol/l
Prothrombin time	14 seconds
APTT	30.1 seconds
Total cholesterol	2.2 mmol/l
HDL cholesterol	0.39 mmol/l

Questions

1. List the abnormalities.
2. Provide one possible explanation.

Answers

The abnormalities include:

- Macrocytic anaemia
- Neutrophilia
- Elevated vitamin B_{12}
- Folate deficiency
- Hypokalaemia
- Abnormal liver function test
- Slightly prolonged prothrombin time
- Elevated TSH with a normal free T4

This patient has a long history of alcohol abuse with hepatic cirrhosis and poor nutritional intake. The raised WBC suggests infection. The macrocytic anaemia is due to folate deficiency and the direct toxic effects of alcohol on the bone marrow. The serum total bilirubin is slightly elevated and the disproportionately high percentage of conjugated bilirubin suggests underlying liver disease rather than haemolysis. Aldehyde derived from alcohol can produce haemolysis, but this is unlikely as the haptoglobin levels in this patient are not markedly reduced. Vitamin B_{12} is stored in the liver (1 µg/kg) and raised serum levels occur in liver disease, including acute hepatitis, cirrhosis, and hepatoma. The low urea and albumin and prolonged prothrombin time reflect impaired hepatocellular function, but transaminases may remain normal in cirrhotic patients. The elevated TSH with a normal free T4 suggests sick euthyroid syndrome.

Folate deficiency in alcoholics is due to:

- Poor dietary intake
- Impaired absorption. Dietary folate exists mainly as polyglutamates, which are converted to monoglutamates before absorption can take place. Alcohol inhibits the intestinal enzyme pterolyglutamate hydrolase that hydrolyses dietary polyglutamate to monoglutamate.
- Impaired folate storage in the liver

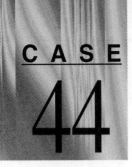

C A S E
44

CASE 44

This is a 75 gram oral glucose tolerance test (OGTT).

Time (min)	Plasma glucose (mmol/l)
0	6.8
30	10.3
60	9.6
90	8.3
120	7.2

Question

What is the diagnosis?

Answer

This patient has Impaired Fasting Glucose (IFG).

In June 2000 Diabetes UK lowered the cut off point for diagnosing diabetes using fasting plasma glucose from 7.8 mmol/l to 7.0 mmol/l. Fasting plasma glucose is much easier to use than the 2 hour long, 75 gram oral glucose tolerance test (OGTT). However, fasting plasma glucose measurement may miss some cases of diabetes and Impaired Glucose Tolerance, which would have been picked up if a glucose tolerance test had been used.

Fasting Plasma Glucose (mmol/l) Diagnostic Criteria

≤ 6	≥ 6.1 and < 7.0	≥ 7.0
Normal	Impaired Fasting Glucose	Diabetes Mellitus

75 gram OGTT: 2 hour Plasma Glucose (mmol/l) Diagnostic Criteria

≤ 7.8	≥ 7.8 and < 11.1 (& fasting < 7)	≥ 11.1
Normal	Impaired Glucose Tolerance	Diabetes Mellitus

Summary of Diabetes UK Recommendations for Diagnosing Diabetes Mellitus

1. In people with symptoms (thirst, polydipsia, polyuria and weight loss) diabetes mellitus is suggested by any one of the following:
   - random plasma glucose ≥ 11.1 mmol/l
   - fasting plasma glucose ≥ 7.0 mmol/l
   - 2 hour plasma glucose ≥ 11.1 mmol/l after 75 gram OGTT
2. In asymptomatic people two abnormal plasma glucose (= any combination of random, fasting, or 2 hour samples) taken on different days are needed for the diagnosis of diabetes mellitus.
3. Impaired Fasting Glucose and Impaired Glucose Tolerance are risk factors for cardiovascular disease and future diabetes. These individuals should receive advice on lifestyle modification (i.e. diet, weight, and exercise) and have other cardiovascular risk factors assessed (i.e. smoking, blood pressure and cholesterol).

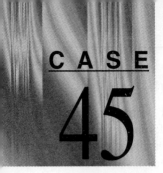

C A S E

45

CASE 45

This is the 75 gram oral glucose tolerance test (OGTT) of a 76-year-old man with headache and visual loss.

Time (min)	Plasma glucose (mmol/l)	Growth hormone (mU/l)
0	5.0	6.4
30	8.2	4.5
60	7.8	21.3
90	6.9	11.8
120	7.3	5.2

Question
What is the diagnosis?

Answer

This patient has acromegaly. In normal subjects glucose administration will suppress growth hormone (GH) release. Failure to suppress GH to less than 2 mU/l at some point during the 2 hours after a 75 gram glucose load is suggestive of acromegaly. In some patients with acromegaly there may be a paradoxical rise in GH levels after a glucose load. The OGTT in acromegaly may also show impaired glucose tolerance or diabetes. Elevated levels of insulin like growth factor 1 (IGF-1) reflect excessive GH secretion and can be used as a screening test for acromegaly. Measurement of IGF-1 is easier to perform than the OGTT. The IGF-1 result should be compared with age and sex match values.

Acromegaly

Acromegaly is the result of excess growth hormone (GH) production by a pituitary adenoma. The annual incidence of acromegaly in the UK population is 3-4 cases per million and the prevalence is 40 cases per million. The treatment of choice is a transphenoidal resection, but bulky tumours with suprasellar extension may require a craniotomy. Radiotherapy is useful if pituitary surgery is inadvisable, or if the excess GH production persists after surgery. However, GH normalises very slowly after irradiation and in these patients GH production could be suppressed by somatostatin analogues such as Octreotide or Lanreotide. All patients given pituitary irradiation should undergo regular endocrine review, because hypopituitarism is common and eventually develops in 50% of these patients within 5 years of radiotherapy.

One of the differential diagnoses of acromegaly is Touraine-Solenti-Gole syndrome (pachydermoperiostosis), which is a familial condition, and growth hormone levels are normal. The features of this syndrome are coarse facial features, finger clubbing, and periosteal bone formation.

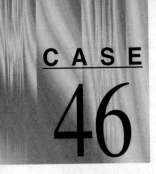

CASE 46

A 72-year-old woman complained of tiredness. She has primary hypothyroidism and was taking 150 µg of thyroxine a day. The following thyroid function tests that were taken at a recent clinic visit.

TSH	22.6 mU/l
Free T4	19.6 pmol/l

Question

What is the explanation for these values?

Answer

The high TSH with normal free T4 in any patient taking thyroxine replacement therapy suggests non-compliance. Failure to take thyroxine leads to a rise in TSH to hypothyroid levels. Restarting thyroxine medication a few weeks before the clinic visit will produce a normal free T4, but the elevated TSH will take much longer to normalise.

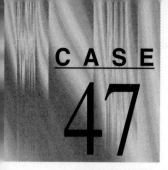

C A S E
47

CASE 47

These are the arterial blood gases of a 64-year-old man with breathlessness. He is receiving 28% oxygen.

pH	7.40
PaO_2	6.2 kPa
$PaCO_2$	7.8 kPa
HCO_3	35.3 mmol/l
Base excess	+ 8.8
Oxygen saturation	82.2%

Question

What is the diagnosis?

Answer

Chronic respiratory acidosis. This man has type 2 respiratory failure due to severe COPD. Renal retention of bicarbonate restores the pH to normal. The Flenley acid base nomogram (see below) is a useful tool for assessing complex respiratory and metabolic disturbance.

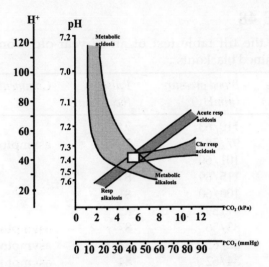

C A S E

48

CASE 48

This is the tilt table test of an 87-year-old woman with unexplained blackouts.

Time (min)	Blood pressure (mmHg)	Pulse (beats/min)	Comments
0	110/63	71	
3	97/58	79	asymptomatic
6	101/60	80	
9	115/69	84	
12	100/60	81	
15	91/59	85	
18	83/56	87	asymptomatic
21	82/65	83	asymptomatic
24	84/62	84	asymptomatic
27	86/57	82	asymptomatic
30	80/54	87	asymptomatic
33	77/53	86	asymptomatic
36	78/52	81	asymptomatic
39	52/38	80	syncope

Question
What is the diagnosis?

Answer

This patient has type 3 vasodepressor syncope.

Vasovagal Syncope

Recurrent unexplained syncope is a common clinical problem. Tilt table testing is widely used to evaluate these patients. Within 10 seconds of standing, 500-1,000 ml of blood is translocated from the thorax to the legs. After 10 minutes of standing up to 700 ml of plasma volume is translocated into the interstitial spaces. The autonomic nervous system operates to counter the inevitable drop in blood pressure induced by taking an upright posture. Vasoconstriction in the skin, muscles, renal and splanchnic circulation is mediated by baroreceptors in the aortic arch and carotid sinus, followed in turn by CNS activation and increased efferent sympathetic outflow. Hormonal responses are slower and involve the renin angiotensin system. These protective mechanisms inexplicably fail in some individuals, who may also demonstrate inappropriate neurally mediated vasodilatation or bradycardia. Asystole for 6 seconds or a drop in systolic blood pressure to 60 mmHg would be sufficient to produce syncope in most adults.

After a pre-tilt period of 5 minutes if there is no venous cannulation, and at least 20 minutes when cannulation is undertaken, the patient is placed at a tilt angle of 60 – 70 degrees for up to a maximum of 45 minutes. If there is no response after 20 minutes of head up tilt, sublingual GTN 400 µg may be given and is followed by another 20 minutes of observation. A positive tilt test is the induction of syncope, which may be accompanied by variable combinations of bradycardia and hypotension. These haemodynamic responses to head up tilt allow vasovagal syncope to be classified into 3 main groups and determine the most appropriate treatment. Patients who have bradycardic responses to head up tilt may benefit from cardiac pacing. Pure forms of vasodepressor syncope are more difficult to treat and therapeutic options include withdrawing blood pressure lowering medication and the use of agents that expand the blood volume.

Classification of positive responses to tilt testing
European Society of Cardiology, Task Force Report 2001*

Type 1:	Mixed	HR falls at time of syncope but not < 40/min *Or* HR falls < 40/min for < 10 seconds, ± < 3 seconds asystole. BP falls before HR falls.
Type 2A:	Cardioinhibitory without asystole	HR < 40/min for > 10 seconds but asystole > 3 seconds does not occur. BP falls before HR falls.
Type 2B:	Cardioinhibitory with asystole	Asystole occurs for > 3 seconds. BP falls coincides with or occurs before HR fall.
Type 3:	Vasodepressor	HR does not fall by > 10% from its peak at time of syncope.

HR = heart rate; BP = Blood Pressure
*Classification of positive responses to tilt testing, European Society of Cardiology, Task Force Report, European Heart Journal 2001: 22; 1256-1306.

CASE 49

A 49-year-old healthy woman was found to have a raised serum calcium. She was asymptomatic and physical examination was unremarkable. Her sister had undergone a subtotal parathyroidectomy for hypercalcaemia.

FBC	normal
CRP	< 8 mg/l
Na	137 mmol/l
K	4.3 mmol/l
Urea	7.4 mmol/l
Creatinine	84 µmol/l
Albumin	36 g/l
Globulin	34 g/l
ALP	118 U/l
ALT	21 U/l
Corrected calcium	2.79 mmol/l
Magnesium	1.3 mmol/l
PTH	5.4 pmol/l (ref 1.6 – 6.9)
TSH	4.88 mU/l
Urine calcium	1.1 mmol/24 h (ref 2.5 –7.5)

Question

What is the most likely diagnosis?

Answer

The most likely diagnosis is familial hypocalciuric hypercalcaemia (FHH). FHH is inherited as an autosomal dominant disorder. Affected individuals with FHH are heterozygous for a mutation in the calcium-sensing receptor (CaSR) gene located on chromosome 3 or 19. The inactivating mutation in the CaSR impairs sensitivity to calcium. As a consequence higher plasma calcium levels are needed to suppress PTH secretion from the parathyroid glands. Impaired sensitivity of the CaSR increases the absorption of calcium and magnesium from the renal tubules. The essential features of FHH are:

- Modest hypercalcaemia (up to 3 mmol/l)
- Relatively low urinary calcium
- Serum magnesium may be elevated
- Inappropriately normal or slightly high PTH levels
- No risk of renal stones, but chondrocalcinosis and pancreatitis are possible associations
- The hypercalcaemia in FHH does not respond to parathyroidectomy.
- A careful search of family members for hypercalcaemia is recommended.

Urinary calcium excretion is dependent on dietary calcium intake. The reference value is 2.5 – 7.5 mmol per day. The following indices are used for quantifying the degree of hypercalciuria:

- urine calcium-creatinine ratio is based on measuring calcium and creatinine in a random urine sample:

$$\frac{\text{urine calcium (mmol/l)}}{\text{urine creatinine (mmol/l)}}$$

The reference range for urine calcium-creatinine ratio is 0.06 – 0.45.

- calcium-creatinine clearance ratio is based on the following items derived from random blood and urine samples:

$$\frac{\text{urine calcium (mmol/l) x serum creatinine (mmol/l)}}{\text{serum calcium (mmo/l) x urine creatinine (mmol/l)}}$$

In primary hyperparathyroidism the calcium-creatinine clearance ratio is > 0.02, whereas in FHH it is < 0.01. However, this ratio lacks specificity.

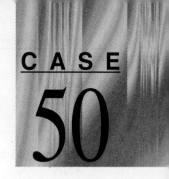

C A S E
50

CASE 50

An 80-year-old man was admitted for investigation of worsening breathlessness over the last sixteen months. He used to be an office worker and gave up smoking 10 years ago. His current medications were: furosemide 40 mg od, perindopril 2 mg od, amiodarone 200 mg od, warfarin, isosorbide mononitrate 20 mg bd, and inhalers (Combivent, Serevent, Becloforte). On examination, he was breathless at rest, and widespread fine crackles could be heard throughout both lungs. Temperature 36.2° Celsius, Pulse 80 bpm (AF), and BP 136/68 mmHg. Heart sounds were normal.

Past medical history

1991   Post-nasal drip and nasal polyps.
       Nasal polypectomy was performed.
1995   Angina and Asthma.
       ECHO showed dilated left ventricle and an ejection fraction 43%.
       FEV1 = 2.55 litre (98% predicted). FVC = 3.34 litres (97% predicted)
       Diuretics and ACE-I were started
2000   AF and LVF were diagnosed. Warfarin and amiodarone were started.

Investigations in 2002

Na	138 mmol/l
K	4.1 mmol/l
Urea	4.1 mmol/l
Creatinine	92 µmol/l
Glucose	5.5 mmol/l
INR	2.7

Hb	10.8 g/dl
WBC	12.9 x 10^9/l
Platelets	567 x 10^9/l
LFT	normal
TSH	4.49 mU/l
Rheumatoid factor	77 U/ml (ref 0-40)
ANA	negative
ECG	AF and RBBB
CXR	widespread interstitial shadowing

Arterial blood gases (on air):

pH	7.43
PaO_2	7.09 kPa
$PaCO_2$	5.53 kPa
HCO_3	26.7 mmol/l
Oxygen saturation	87.8%

Lung Function Test in 2002

		Predicted	Observed	% Predicted
FEV1	L	2.45	1.54	62
FVC	L	3.31	1.74	52
FEV1/FVC	%	73	88	120
RV	L	2.74	1.37	50
TLC	L	6.42	3.35	52
RV/TLC	%	45	41	91
DLCO		7.46	2.41	32
VA		5.46	2.44	44
KCO		1.16	0.99	85

Question
What is the diagnosis?

Answer

Amiodarone Induced Pulmonary Toxicity.

Amiodarone is an iodinated benzofuran class III antiarrhythmic agent that is used for a wide range of supraventricular and ventricular arrhythmias. Its side effects include skin pigmentation, photosensitivity, corneal deposits, thyroid dysfunction, bone marrow disease, and pulmonary toxicity. The incidence of amiodarone induced pulmonary disease is around 5-10% when the drug is used in high doses (> 400 mg a day), and 1-2% for patients receiving smaller doses.

Types of Amiodarone Induced Pulmonary Toxicity (AIPT)

Amiodarone can produce the following respiratory problems:
* Interstitial pneumonitis-fibrosis
* Acute Respiratory Distress Syndrome
* Bronchiolitis Obliterans with Organising Pneumonia
* Solitary pulmonary mass
* Pleural effusion ± pericardial effusion

Mechanisms of AIPT

* Pneumonitis describes the potentially reversible inflammatory process that responds to corticosteroids, which is followed by irreversible fibrosis, especially if the drug has not been withdrawn in time.
* Amiodarone inhibits lysosomal phospholipase, leading to the accumulation of phospholipids, which are directly toxic to lung tissues.
* Immune injury by CD8 T-cell lymphocytes.

Risk Factors for AIPT

* Dose of amiodarone received
* Duration of amiodarone treatment. AIPT can develop after cessation of amiodarone therapy, due to its long half-life in lung tissues.
* Chest infection
* Oxygen therapy
* Open heart surgery

Clinical Features of AIPT

- Onset of symptoms can be abrupt or insidious
- Fever
- Non-productive cough
- Dyspnoea with hypoxaemia that is often out of all proportion to the chest X-ray signs.
- Pleuritic chest pain
- Diffuse crackles and pleural rub

Diagnostic Tests

- Chest X-ray will show one of these common radiological patterns of AIPT: diffuse interstitial infiltrates, pleural effusion, or solitary mass.
- Lung function tests typically demonstrate a restrictive defect and impaired gas transfer coefficient. A restrictive defect may not be apparent in patients with pre-existing chronic bronchitis and emphysema.
- Gallium lung scan. Gallium-67 isotope will show an active inflammatory process in lung tissues, but is now replaced by high resolution chest CT scan (HRCT).
- HRCT shows a diffuse ground glass appearance, indicating pneumonitis.
- Open lung biopsy will show fibrous thickening of the interstitium with lymphocytic and plasma cell infiltration; foamy macrophages in the alveoli; and bronchiolitis obliterans with organising pneumonia (BOOP).

Treatment of AIPT

- Supportive therapy for respiratory failure and infection
- Stop amiodarone. If life threatening arrhythmias render this strategy impossible, reduce the dose of amiodarone and add corticosteroids.
- Corticosteroids are needed for many months due to the long elimination half-life of amiodarone. Typical initial doses of prednisolone are 40-60mg daily, which are reduced gradually over several months. Relapse may occur if corticosteroids are withdrawn too quickly.
- Monitor response to corticosteroids with repeat HRCT

Drugs Associated with Pulmonary Fibrosis

- Antiarrhythmics (amiodarone, flecainide, practolol, lignocaine)
- Cytotoxic agents (azathioprine, methotrexate, cyclophosphamide, busulfan, bleomycin, mitomycin)
- Anti-inflammatory agents (gold, penicillamine)
- Antibiotics (sulfasalazine, nitrofurantoin)
- Anticonvulsants (phenytoin, carbamazepine)
- Pesticide (paraquat)
- Others (methysergide, high dose oxygen)

N.B. Many of these agents also produce bronchiolitis obliterans with organising pneumonia (BOOP), in which granulation tissue is found in both bronchiolar lumen and alveolar spaces.

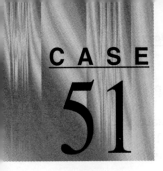

C A S E
51

CASE 51

A 75-year-old was admitted to hospital with an unexplained blackout. Her husband saw her get up from a chair to answer the doorbell when she suddenly lost consciousness. In the previous 6 months she has had recurrent dizziness induced by standing and 'fainted' on a number of occasions. She was a life long non-smoker and did not drink alcohol. The only medication taken was co-proxamol for chronic back pain. On examination, the temperature was 36° Celsius, pulse 70 bpm regular, supine BP 139/85 mmHg and 110/60 mmHg on standing. The rest of the physical examination was unremarkable.

Na	140 mmol/l
K	4.3 mmol/l
Urea	8 mmol/l
Creatinine	119 µmol/l
Hb	12.5 g/dl
WBC	4.6 x 10⁹/l
Platelets	201 x 10⁹/l
LFT	normal
TSH	normal
CXR	normal
ECG	normal

Autonomic Function Tests

BP supine	120/70mmHg
BP after 2 minutes standing	80/70 mmHg

Cold pressor test (ice water immersion for 1 min) (normal response = 10 mmHg rise in systolic and diastolic BP)
- change in systolic BP = + 2 mmHg
- change in diastolic BP = 0 mmHg

Valsalva Ratio   1.0   (abnormal ≤ 1.0 for 70y old)
    (forced expiration 15 sec)
Heart rate change with respiration 0   (abnormal < 7 for 70y old)
    (I-E difference)
Heart rate change on standing   1.0   (abnormal ≤ 1.0 for 70y old)
    (30:15 ratio)

Short Synacthen Test

Plasma cortisol before and after 250 µg Synacthen IV
0 min cortisol   272 nmol/l
30 min cortisol   673 nmol/l

Noradrenaline (norepinephrine) levels

Supine	0.6 nmol/l (normal supine = 0.65 – 3.84)
After 2 min standing	1.1 nmol/l (normal standing = 1.18 – 6.50)
After 5 min standing	1.3 nmol/l
After 10 min standing	1.4 nmol/l

Question
What is the diagnosis?

Answer

This patient has Pure Autonomic Failure (PAF), which used to be called Idiopathic Orthostatic Hypotension. There is severe postural (orthostatic) hypotension and the autonomic function tests show no variability in heart rate in response to respiration, standing, and Valsalva manoeuvre. In PAF supine levels of noradrenaline are low and suggest a peripheral lesion in the autonomic pathway.

The Clinical Features of Autonomic Failure

- Cardiovascular (postural hypotension)
- Cutaneous (anhidrosis)
- Gastrointestinal (gastroparesis, constipation, diarrhoea)
- Genitourinary (urinary frequency, nocturia, retention of urine, erectile dysfunction)
- Eye (Horner's syndrome, visual obscurations)
- Respiratory (sleep apnoea, stridor)
- Central nervous system (Parkinson's disease, cerebellar or pyramidal signs)

The Classification of Autonomic Failure

Primary autonomic failure

- Pure autonomic failure (PAF). In PAF there is no other neurodegenerative disorder.
- Shy-Drager Syndrome (SDS) is also called Multiple System atrophy (MSA) and refers to autonomic failure in association with other neurodegenerative disorders such as Parkinson's disease, cerebeller ataxia, pyramidal signs, or mixture of these.

Secondary autonomic failure

- Central brain lesions, especially vascular lesions, tumour, or demyelination, in the hypothalamus and midbrain
- Spinal cord lesions: transverse myelitis, syringobulbia or syringomyelia, tumours
- Peripheral lesions: Guillain-Barré syndrome, tabes dorsalis, diabetes, amyloid, autoimmune disease, alcohol, HIV, prion disease
- Age-related autonomic failure
- Drugs, especially antidepressants and antihypertensives.

Testing the Integrity of the Baroreceptor Reflex Arc

Heart rate and blood pressure are controlled by the baroreceptor reflex arc which consists of the following elements:

- An afferent loop is made up of the stretch receptors in the carotid sinus and aortic arch that detect changes in blood pressure and convey this information to the brain;
- The vasomotor control centre of the brain and cortico-hypothalamic centres;
- An efferent loop consists of the parasympathetic vagal innervation of the heart and the sympathetic outflow from the spinal cord and sympathetic ganglia to the resistance blood vessels and myocardium.

The overall integrity of this baroreceptor reflex arc is tested by:

- Heart rate and BP responses to standing
- Heart rate and BP responses during the Valsalva manoeuvre

The sympathetic and parasympathetic efferent pathways can be tested separately:

- Sympathetic pathway. The rise in blood pressure in response to the cold pressor test, mental stress (serial 7's), isometric exercise (during sustained hand grip at 30% maximum strength). Fluorodopamine positron emission tomography can show the loss of sympathetic nerves in the myocardium in patient with PAF (NEJM 1997;336:696-702). In SDS/MSA these sympathetic fibres are intact.
- Parasympathetic pathway. The change in heart rate in response to deep respiration (6 breaths per minute) or immersion of the face in water (dive reflex).

An ECG machine that provides a continuous paper trace is used to record these rapid changes in heart rate. For a description of the methodology consult Ewing, DJ and Clarke, BF. Diagnosis and management of diabetic autonomic neuropathy. BMJ 1982;285:916-18. Age related abnormal low scores for these tests are quoted by Wieling, W. (1996) Laboratory assessment of disturbances in cardiovascular control. In: Kenny, RA (ed), Syncope in the older patient. Chapman and Hall, London, pp 47-71.

Noradrenaline Levels

- Supine levels of noradrenaline are lower than normal in PAF and suggest a peripheral autonomic lesion.
- Supine levels of noradrenaline is normal or slightly elevated in SDS/MSA
- The rise in noradrenaline on standing is attenuated in both PAF and SDS/MSA

Treatment of Orthostatic Hypotension

Non-pharmacological

- Avoid large meals, alcohol, vasoactive medication. An hour after meals there is a drop in blood pressure, probably due to splanchnic dilatation, and this is more likely to occur with meals rich in simple carbohydrates.
- Postural training: 20 cm head up tilt at night. Sleeping with the head of the bed raised stimulates the renin-angiotensin system, encourages fluid retention and volume expansion, and raises blood pressure.
- Compression hosiery and abdominal binders reduce venous pooling of blood in the lower limbs, increase venous return to the heart, and reduce falls in blood pressure.
- Physical manoeuvres: crossing the legs increases peripheral vascular resistance and reduces the drop in blood pressure induced by standing (Lancet 1992;339:897-98)

Pharmacological

- Sympathomimetic/vasoconstrictive agents: ephedrine, clonidine, phenylephrine, pindolol, caffeine, ergot
- Tyramine and MAO-A inhibitor (Bovril 12 gram tds and moclobemide 150 mg tds). Tyramine releases noradrenaline from nerve endings. Approximately 90% of the tyramine from the diet is inactivated by MAO-B enzyme in the gut wall. The remaining 10% is inactivated by the liver's MAO-A enzyme. Moclobemide is a selective MAO-A inhibitor which allows this 10% portion of dietary tyramine to become available to the nervous system, where it releases noradrenaline and produces a pressor effect (Lancet 1994;344:1263-5).
- Salt and water retention induced by fludrocortisone, DDAVP, or NSAID.

CASE 52

A 72-year-old retired policeman suffered from intermittent fainting attacks and blackouts for several years and lost his car licence. Investigations at previous hospitals included normal Holter monitoring, EEG, echocardiogram, and CT brain scan. Physical examination was unrewarding. There was no evidence of postural hypotension. The following ECG tracing showed the response to right carotid sinus massage.

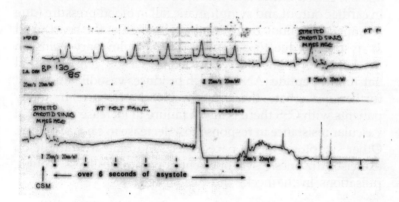

A VVI permanent cardiac pacemaker was inserted. He felt well for several months and his driving licence was returned to him. Then at a routine clinic visit he complained of breathlessness with the recurrence of blackouts. His pacemaker was checked and found to be working normally.

Questions
1. What is the cause of this man's original blackouts?
2. What is the most likely cause of his latest symptoms?

Answers

1. This man has carotid sinus syncope (CSS), which is also called carotid sinus hypersensitivity or carotid sinus syndrome.
2. Pacemaker syndrome.

CSS is an important and treatable cause of unexplained falls, dizziness and syncope, especially in the elderly. This patient was given a "VVI" type of cardiac pacemaker. Ventricular pacing may produce the pacemaker syndrome in the patients with CSS or vasovagal syncope. During VVI pacing, ventriculoatrial conduction, i.e. retrograde fashion along the atrioventricular node, allows electrical stimuli from the pacemaker to activate the atria. In this way ventricular systole occurs at the same time as atrial contraction, a phenomenon called atrioventricular dyssynchrony. Atrial contraction against closed mitral and tricuspid valves leads to: 1) a drop in cardiac output and symptomatic fall in blood pressure (due to impaired venous return to the right side of the heart); and 2) dyspnoea (due to distension of the pulmonary veins on the left side of the heart). Atrial distension releases atrial natriuretic peptide (ANP), which produces vasodilatation and further exacerbate the drop in blood pressure. In many patients with CSS there is also a failure to increase peripheral vascular resistance in response to a decrease in cardiac output. Other symptoms of the pacemaker syndrome are: fatigue on exercise, dizziness, syncope, chest pain or fullness, cough, pulsations in the neck, and headache.

The diagnosis of pacemaker syndrome is often difficult, because of the vague nature of these symptoms and their obvious similarity to the original cardiac symptoms prior to pacemaker implantation. Cannon 'a' waves, or a ≥ 20 mmHg drop in systolic blood pressure during cardiac pacing with reproduction of symptoms will support the diagnosis of pacemaker syndrome. Upgrading to a dual chamber pacemaker ("DDI" or "DDD") that restores the normal sequence of atrial and ventricular contraction will eliminate these symptoms.

Pacemaker Code

British Pacing and Electrophysiology Group (BPEG) Pacemaker Code

Position of letter	I	II	III	IV	V
	Chamber (s) paced	Chamber (s) sensed	Response to sensing	Program rate modulation	Anti-tachycardia function (s)
	A = Atrium	A = Atrium	T = Triggered	P = Simple Programmable	P = Pacing
	V = Ventricle	V = Ventricle	I = Inhibited	M = Multiprogram	S = Shock
	D = Dual (A+V)	D = Dual (A+V)	D = Dual (T+I)	C= communicating	D = Dual (P+S)
	0 = None	0 = None	0 = None	0 = None	0 = None
				R = Rate modulation	

Carotid Sinus Syncope

The incidence of CSS increases with age and one in 10 elderly people can be shown to have carotid hypersensitivity. However, only about 0.5% of the elderly population will have spontaneous symptoms. (The aetiology of CSS is discussed by O'Mahony, D. Pathophysiology of carotid sinus hypersensitivity in elderly patients. Lancet 1995:346: 950-952.)

Carotid Sinus Massage

With the patient lying supine apply a 5 second massage at the level of the upper border of the thyroid cartilage. Right and left carotids are tested separately with a 30 second interval between the two sides. If negative, repeating the test procedure with the patient in an upright position. The responses to carotid sinus massage are classified into:

- Cardioinhibitory type is an asystole of $\geq$ 3 seconds. The treatment is cardiac pacing, preferably DDI or DDD.
- Vasodepressor type is a fall in systolic blood pressure of $\geq$ 50 mmHg. The treatment is often unsatisfactory. Try vasoconstrictors like ephedrine and ergot, but these are often poorly tolerated. Fludrocortisone may also help as it sensitises adrenoreceptors to circulating catecholamines.
- Mixed type. To evaluate the vasodepressor component of the response, giving 600 µg of atropine IV before repeating the massage can abolish the cardioinhibitory component. Treatment is cardiac pacing and medications to reduce vasodilation.

Asystole occurs on average at 2 seconds into the carotid sinus massage. The maximum drop in blood pressure occurs on average at 18 seconds.

Contraindications to carotid sinus massage are:
- Carotid bruits
- Recent MI (within 3 months)
- Recent stroke (within 3 months)
- Previous VT or VF

The incidence of complications was 7 neurological problems in 5,000 massage episodes (0.14%), including transient visual field defect (n = 2), dysphasia (n = 1) or limb weakness (n = 4) (Munro NC et al. Incidence of complications after carotid sinus massage in older patients with syncope. JAGS 1994; 42:1248-51.)

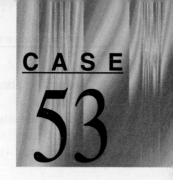
CASE 53

This 72-year-old woman is breathless at rest. She is taking
bendroflumethiazide 5 mg od for hypertension.

Arterial blood gases (on air):

pH	7.49
PaO_2	8.5 kPa
$PaCO_2$	5.5 kPa
HCO_3	31.3 mmol/l
Base excess	+ 7.2
Oxygen saturation	93%
Na	133 mmol/l
K	3.2 mmol/l
Urea	4.9 mmol/l
Creatinine	77 µmol/l
Glucose	7.8 mmol/l

Question

What are the 3 possible diagnoses?

Answer

1. Metabolic alkalosis secondary to thiazide induced hypokalaemia.
2. Uncompensated respiratory alkalosis.
3. Type 1 respiratory failure, which occurs in chest infection, pneumonia, or pulmonary embolism.

CASE 54

An 84-year-old woman with rheumatoid arthritis has been breathless at rest for about 2 months. The respiratory rate was 40 per minute, but there were no other abnormalities on physical examination. Her PEFR and chest X-ray were normal. These are her arterial blood gases taken on room air:

pH	7.62
PaO_2	13.1 kPa
$PaCO_2$	2.1 kPa
HCO_3	15.5 mmol/l
Base excess	- 3.7
Oxygen saturation	98.3%

Questions

1. What is the diagnosis?
2. What other investigations are needed?

Answers

1. Acute respiratory alkalosis
2. Serum electrolytes
   Plasma salicylate level to exclude aspirin poisoning

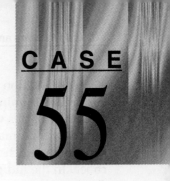

C A S E

55

CASE 55

A 17-year-old man was admitted to hospital for investigation. Over a period of 2 months he has had cramp like central abdominal pain, watery diarrhoea alternating with constipation, and 8 kg weight loss. He was not taking any regular medications. Family and past medical histories were unremarkable. On examination, he looked thin (BMI = 15), pulse 80 bpm, BP 120/60 mmHg, and temperature 36° Celsius. There was tenderness over the right iliac fossa and suprapubic area.

Hb	12.6 g/dl
WBC	9.3 x 10⁹/l
Platelets	623 x 10⁹/l
MCV	74.9 fl
CRP	79 mg/l
Na	137 mmol/l
K	4.5 mmol/l
Urea	3.0 mmol/l
Creatinine	78 µmol/l
Albumin	27 g/l
Globulin	32 g/l
Bilirubin	5 µmol/l
ALP	78 U/l
ALT	7 U/l
AST	16 U/l
Glucose	7.1 mmol/l
Amylase	52 U/l
Gliadin IgA	2 U/ml (ref 0-16)
Gliadin IgG	9 U/ml (ref 0-43)
Transglutaminase IgG	1 U/ml (ref 0-5)
CXR	normal
Abdominal X-ray	normal

Questions
1. What is the most likely diagnosis?
2. What is the differential diagnosis?

Answers

The combination of a high CRP, anaemia with a low MCV, and hypoalbuminaemia suggests inflammatory bowel disease as a cause of this young man's gastrointestinal symptoms. The inflammatory markers would be normal in malabsorption syndromes such as coeliac disease and pancreatic steatorrhoea. In the indigenous UK population the most likely cause for these symptoms is Crohn's disease. However, patients presenting with these symptoms who live elsewhere in the world will have a larger number of other conditions in the differential diagnosis (see below).

Crohn's Disease

Crohn's disease is a chronic inflammatory disorder of unknown aetiology that can affect any part of the gastrointestinal tract from the mouth to anus and the course of the disease is marked by recurrent relapses. The peak age of onset is 15-30 years with another smaller peak at 60-80 years. The prevalence is 50 per 100,000 of the population and incidence 3-6 per 100,000. It is slightly commoner in males. The bowel lesion of Crohn's disease is characterised by transmural inflammation, i.e. affecting all layers of the bowel wall, with non-caseating granulomas. This inflammatory process leads to:

- Obstructive symptoms initially from inflammatory strictures and then fibrotic lesions
- Fistulae into other organs, e.g. colon, bladder, vagina
- Adhesions
- Abscess formation
- Malabsorption

Common Symptoms in Crohn's Disease

- Diarrhoea is non-bloody - except in colonic involvement (i.e. Crohn's colitis). Crohn's colitis presents with bloody diarrhoea and perianal disease (anal fissures and abscesses)
- Steatorrhoea is due to small bowel disease and malabsorption
- Obstructive symptoms including intermittent cramping abdominal pain and bloating

- Weight loss
- Vomiting
- Fever
- Right iliac fossa mass in ileocaecal disease
- In children there is growth failure and delayed puberty

Extra-intestinal Manifestations of Crohn's Disease

There are also many extra-intestinal (i.e. occurring outside the bowel) manifestations, including:
- Oral aphthous ulcers
- Cutaneous (erythema nodosum, pyoderma gangrenosum)
- Monoarthritis (usually larger joints such as knee or ankle)
- Sacroiliitis and ankylosing spondylitis
- Ocular (episcleritis, iritis, uveitis)
- Hepatic (fatty liver, pericholangitis, sclerosing cholangitis, chronic active hepatitis, cirrhosis – but all these are much more common in ulcerative colitis)
- Gallstones
- Renal (stones, amyloidosis)

Differential Diagnosis of Crohn's Disease

Crohn's disease usually affects the ileocolic regions and this is reflected by the wide differential diagnosis, which includes:
- Ulcerative colitis
- Ileocaecal tuberculosis
- Appendicitis
- Amoebic colitis
- Systemic vasculitis
- Yersinia enterocolitica infection
- Carcinoid tumour
- Gut lymphoma
- Behçet's disease
- HIV disease
- In females the differential diagnosis would include endometriosis and ovarian pathology

Investigations in Crohn's disease
- Inflammatory markers (ESR, CRP, WBC) will be raised
- Anaemia in Crohn's disease has many possible factors: blood loss, iron malabsorption in small bowel disease,

vitamin B_{12} malabsorption in ileal disease, or the "anaemia of chronic disease"

- Low serum albumin reflects protein losing enteropathy, malabsorption, and poor oral intake
- Stool cultures will be negative
- In Crohn's disease antibodies to the yeast *Saccharomyces cerevisiae* (ASCA) is positive and P-ANCA is negative. In contrast, ASCA is usually negative and P-ANCA positive in ulcerative colitis.
- Barium studies of the upper gastrointestinal tract. Small bowel follow through will show disease of the terminal ileum, including the following characteristic signs: narrowing (string sign of Kantor), deep 'rose-thorn' ulceration (yielding a "cobblestone" appearance), and "skip lesions" (disease areas separated by normal bowel).
- Barium enema will show colonic involvement and fistulae.
- Colonoscopy may show aphthous ulcers
- CT or MRI of the abdomen is used to evaluate inflammatory mass or abscess
- Radionuclide scans can demonstrate the extent of bowel inflammation, but is reserved for patients who are too ill for barium studies or colonoscopy.

Treatment of Crohn's Disease

- Elemental diets may induce remission in small bowel disease. In some patients the diarrhoea may be due to lactase deficiency.
- Steroids. Prednisolone (40 mg od) can induce remission in acute disease, and the dose should be tailed off as quickly as possible. Steroids are not used for maintenance therapy in view of the long term side effects. Azathioprine is used if there are difficulties with withdrawal of steroids. Severe disease will require admission to hospital for IV steroids, fluids, and parenteral nutrition. Avoid opiate antidiarrhoeal agents in patients with acute Crohn's colitis, as there is a risk of precipitating toxic megacolon.
- Sulfasalazine (orally or in form of enemata) is useful in Crohn's colitis, but does not maintain remission and is of no help in small bowel disease.

- Antibiotics (metronidazole, ciprofloxacin, or co-trimoxazole) are useful in perianal disease and intra-abdominal abscess.
- Anti-tumour necrosis factor (TNF) antibody. TNF is thought to play an important role in the inflammatory process. Infliximab is a chimeric mouse-human monoclonal antibody directed against TNF and may induce remission in Crohn's disease resistant to other treatments, including those patients with refractory perianal disease and fistulae.
- Surgery is reserved for obstruction, toxic megacolon, fistulae, abscess, and perianal disease.

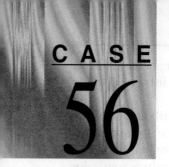

C A S E

56

CASE 56

These are the routine blood results for a 79-year-old man with ulcerative colitis:

Hb	6.7 g/dl
WBC	1.6 x 10⁹/l
Neutrophils	0.4 x 10⁹/l (ref 2-7.5)
Lymphocytes	1.02 x 10⁹/l (ref 1-4)
Platelets	86 x 10⁹/l
MCV	86.1 fl

Question

What is the most likely cause for this blood picture?

Answer

This man is taking mesalazine and azathioprine for his colitis. The diagnostic possibilities are:

- Azathioprine induced neutropenia.
- Mesalazine induced folate deficiency can manifest as a pancytopenia.

Thiopurine Methyltransferase

Thiopurine methyltransferase (TPMT) inactivates azathioprine. Approximately 10% of the population have modestly reduced TPMT enzyme activity and 0.3% have little or no detectable enzyme activity. Both groups are at an increased risk of bone marrow toxicity from azathioprine.

Acquired Causes of Pancytopenia

- Megaloblastic anaemia: vitamin B-12 and folic acid deficiency
- Drugs: chloramphenicol, carbimazole, phenylbutazone, gold, cytotoxic agents.
- Infective: hepatitis viruses, Epstein-Barr virus, HIV, Parvovirus B-19, mycobacteria.
- Toxic chemicals: benzene, insecticides
- Radiation
- Myelodysplastic syndrome
- Myelophthisic anaemia: bone marrow infiltration (myeloma, secondary cancer, leukaemia, lymphoma, myelofibrosis).
- Hypersplenism
- Severe septicaemia
- Paroxysmal nocturnal haemoglobinuria (PNH) is due to an acquired somatic mutation of the PIGA gene on the X-chromosome. This defect in the PIGA (phosphatidylinositol glycan class A) gene impairs the ability to synthesise the glycosyl-phosphatidylinositol (GPI) anchor that binds complement-regulating surface proteins, including decay-accelerating factor (DAF) or CD55, homologous restriction factor (HRF) or C8 binding protein, and membrane inhibitor of reactive lysis (MIRL) or CD59. Absence of these surface proteins renders all haemopoietic cells sensitive to complement mediated lysis. PNH is associated with thrombotic disease, giving rise to hepatic vein occlusion (Budd-Chiari

syndrome), myocardial infarction, and stroke. Thrombosis is due to the deficiency of CD59 on platelet membranes, which leads to platelet aggregation.

- Systemic lupus erythematosus (SLE)
- Thymoma
- Pregnancy

Supportive Treatment of Pancytopenia

Pancytopenia is the most severe form of bone marrow failure and these patients are best managed by haematologists.

- Treat infection: antibiotic (quinolones), anti-viral (acyclovir), anti-fungal (fluconazole or amphotericin). Neutropenic patients (absolute neutrophil count < 1.0 x 10^9/l) are susceptible to a range of gram negative infections, especially Pseudomonas. Early empirical use of antibiotics with activity against gram negative organisms and Pseudomonas (e.g. quinolines such as IV ofloxacin 200mg bd, or IV ceftazidime 2 g tds, or IV imipenem 500mg qds) may reduce episodes of septic shock and mortality. Severely neutropenia patients (neutrophil count of less than 0.5 x 10^9/l) require protective isolation or reverse barrier nursing.
- Consider growth factors such as granulocyte-macrophage colony-stimulating factor, erythropoietin and thrombo–poietin.
- Transfusion for anaemia
- Platelet transfusion only if there is active bleeding

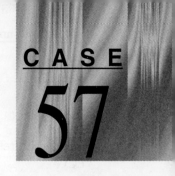

CASE

57

CASE 57

A 65-year-old woman presented with sudden onset visual loss in both eyes. Over the last 3 months she had suffered from epigastric pain and lost 7 kg in weight. She smoked 20 cigarettes a day, but did not drink alcohol. Past medical history included hypertension, which was treated with bendroflume-thiazide 2.5 mg od. On examination, she was emaciated (BMI = 19) and clubbed. There was no lymphadenopathy. She was in atrial fibrillation. The apex heart rate was 120 bpm and BP = 140/80 mmHg. The jugular venous pressure was raised. A systolic murmur was heard at the apex of the heart. The chest was clear on auscultation. There was tender hepatomegaly. Pitting oedema was present up to the level of both knees. The pupils were equal in size and reacted normally to light. The optic fundi were normal. There were no other focal neurological signs. She seemed curiously unconcerned by her inability to visualise her environment.

Hb	10.6 g/dl
WBC	8.1 x 10⁹/l
Platelets	72 x 10⁹/l
CRP	36 mg/l
FDP	1041 µg/ml (ref < 5)
Prothrombin time	27 seconds (ref <13)
APTT	83 seconds (ref < 33)
Fibrinogen	0.7 g/l (ref 2.0-4.5)
Na	132 mmol/l
K	3.3 mmol/l
Urea	12.8 mmol/l
Creatinine	132 µmol/l
Corrected calcium	2.5 mmol/l
Bilirubin	43 µmol/l
ALP	264 U/l

AST	67 U/l
Albumin	28 g/l
Globulin	32 g/l
Urinalysis	2+ blood, protein 2+
MSU	sterile
Blood cultures	sterile
ECG	atrial fibrillation and left ventricular hypertrophy
CXR	cardiomegaly

Question
What are the diagnostic possibilities?

Answer

The diagnostic possibilities are:

1. Nonbacterial thrombotic or "marantic" endocarditis and disseminated intravascular coagulation (DIC) in a patient with an intra-abdominal malignancy. Cortical blindness from bilateral occipital lobe infarction can occur in marantic endocarditis, due to either embolism of sterile fibrin clot from cardiac valves or cerebral thrombosis in DIC.
2. Cortical blindness from cardiogenic embolism to both occipital lobes in a patient with hypertensive heart disease and atrial fibrillation.
3. Bacterial endocarditis is less likely in this patient who has evidence of malignancy and negative blood cultures.

Disseminated Intravascular Coagulation (DIC)

DIC is a state of imbalance between clot formation (mediated by thrombin) and clot lysis (mediated by plasmin). Thrombosis consumes platelets, clotting factors, and the natural anti-coagulants, which consequently become depleted. Thrombin cleaves fibrinogen to produce soluble fibrin monomers and fibrinopeptides A and B. Fibrin monomers associate together under the influence of factor XIII to form cross-linked insoluble fibrin. During clot lysis plasmin cleaves the cross-linked insoluble fibrin to liberate D-dimers and fibrin degradation product (FDPs). Consequently, in DIC too much thrombin activation will promote thrombosis; and too much plasmin formation with depletion of platelets and clotting factors will lead to a haemorrhagic state. Acute forms of DIC are usually haemorrhagic. Chronic DIC usually presents as a prothrombotic state with migratory thrombophlebitis (Trousseau's sign), venous thrombosis, pulmonary embolism, and marantic endocarditis.

DIC is associated with many conditions, including:

- Sepsis
- Major trauma
- Burns
- Malignancy
- Liver disease
- Obstetric complications (placental abruption, amniotic fluid embolism, eclampsia)
- Incompatible blood transfusion

Formation of FDPs and D-dimers

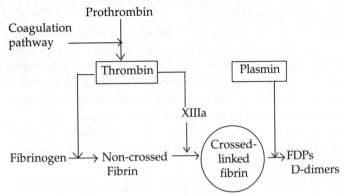

- Snake bites
- Haemolytic uraemic syndrome
- Aortic aneurysms, giant haemangiomas (Kasabach-Merritt syndrome)

There is no specific test for DIC. However, DIC is suggested by the following constellation of haematological abnormalities:

- Thrombocytopenia
- Prolonged clotting times (PT, APTT, thrombin time)
- Low fibrinogen levels
- Elevated levels of D-dimers and fibrin degradation products (FDPs)

Notes:

1. In acute DIC, fibrinogen is reduced by about 50% and clotting times (PT, APTT, TT) are prolonged by about 50%. However, normal values for these tests would not completely exclude DIC.

2. In chronic DIC, fibrinogen and platelet counts may be elevated in response to illness, inflammation, or injury. Clotting times may be shortened due to increased levels of clotting factors.

3. D-dimers (reference range < 0.5 µg/ml) and FDPs (reference range < 5 µg/ml) on their own are not specific tests for DIC.

4. Schistocytes may appear in the blood film and suggest microangiopathic haemolysis by fibrin strands located in blood vessels, but do not provide proof of DIC.

Reference: Baglin T. Disseminated intravascular coagulation: diagnosis and treatment. BMJ 1196:312: 683-7.

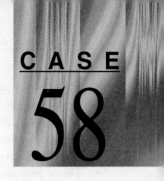

C A S E

58

CASE 58

A previously healthy 46-year-old man was admitted to the CCU with an acute anterior myocardial infarction. He had never smoked cigarettes and was taking no regular medications. His father died suddenly at the age of 40 years with a myocardial infarction. The following fasting lipid profile was obtained 12 hours after admission:

Total cholesterol	10.8 mmol/l
LDL cholesterol	8.8 mmol/l
HDL cholesterol	1.2 mmol/l
Triglycerides	1.5 mmol/l

Question

What is this lipid disorder and describe its associated features?

Answer

This patient has familial hypercholesterolaemia (FH). The clinical features of FH are:

- Autosomal dominant inheritance
- Heterozygous FH affects 1 in 500 of the UK population. Men and women are equally affected
- There are more than 400 mutations in the LDL receptor gene on chromosome 19
- LDL receptor numbers are markedly reduced or non-functional, leading to failure to clear LDL from the circulation
- Total cholesterol is > 7.5 mmol/l in heterozygotes (> 15 mmol/l in homozygotes)
- Triglyceride level is normal
- Eyelid xanthelasmata and premature corneal arcus (i.e. appearing before the age of 30-40 years) are common, but neither are specific for FH
- Tendon xanthomata appear over the knuckles or Achilles tendon. These xanthomata are absent during childhood, but occur with increasing age, and are seen in more than 60% of heterozygous FH by the third decade. However, 20% of patients never develop them.
- In heterozygous FH, there is a 4-fold increase in CHD with symptoms appearing in the fourth decade. Left untreated 60% of patients with heterozygous FH will have had a myocardial infarct by the age of 60 years. Homozygous FH can develop myocardial infarction as early as the first 2 years of life and without aggressive cholesterol lowering treatment survival beyond the age of 30 years is unlikely.
- Heterozygous FH is treated with a statin (HMG CoA reductase) in high dose, often in combination with other cholesterol lowering medications such as bile acid sequestrants.
- Homozygous FH may need plasmapheresis to remove LDL, portacaval shunting, and liver transplantation. Patients with homozygous FH who lack functioning LDL receptors do not respond to statins.

The Diagnosis of Familial Hypercholesterolaemia

At present the diagnosis of familial hypercholesterolaemia is made on the basis of the lipid profile, clinical signs, and family history. Accurate genetic diagnosis is only possible in specialist centres. The following diagnostic criteria are given by the Simon Broome register of familial hypercholesterolaemia.

Definite Familial Hypercholesterolaemia

- Total cholesterol > 7.5 mmol/l in an adult (or LDL cholesterol > 4.9 mmol/l) and
- Tendon xanthoma in the patient or in a first or second degree relative

Possible Familial Hypercholesterolaemia

- Total cholesterol > 7.5 mmol/l in an adult (or LDL cholesterol > 4.9 mmol/l)
  plus a family history of at least one of the following:
- Premature myocardial infarction (i.e. under the age of 60 years old in a first degree relative, or under 50 years old in a second degree relative)
- Hypercholesterolaemia in a first or second degree relative

Reference: Risk of fatal coronary heart disease in familial hypercholesterolaemia. Scientific Steering Committee on behalf of the Simon Broome Register Group. BMJ 1991; 303: 893-6

Genetic Classification of Primary Hyperlipidaemia

Elevated levels of blood lipids can be the result of genetic disorders of lipoprotein metabolism. The genetic classification by Goldstein is much more user friendly than the earlier Fredrickson (WHO) classification. In the genetic classification lipid disorders are grouped into hypertriglyceridaemia alone, hypercholesterolaemia alone, or combined hyperlipidaemia when both triglyceride and cholesterol are elevated.

Hypertriglyceridaemia Alone

- Familial hypertriglyceridaemia (prevalence = 1 in 300) is autosomal dominant. Defect unknown. Eruptive xanthomas, lipaemia retinalis and pancreatitis. Can co-exist with hypercholesterolaemia. Triglyceride levels are exaggerated by obesity, diabetes, alcohol, pregnancy, contraceptive pill, thiazide and corticosteroids.

- Familial lipoprotein lipase deficiency (prevalence = 1 per million) and apoprotein C-II deficiency are both autosomal recessive disorders. High levels of chylomicrons (triglyceride levels > 20 mmol/l) present in childhood with eruptive xanthomas, lipaemia retinalis, retinal vein thrombosis, pancreatitis and hepatosplenomegaly. Fresh frozen plasma lowers triglyceride levels in apoprotein C-II deficiency, but has no effect in lipoprotein deficiency.

Hypercholesterolaemia Alone

- Monogenic heterozygous familial hypercholesterolaemia (prevalence = 1 in 500), or homozygous familial hypercholesterolaemia (prevalence 1 per million).
- Polygenic 'non-familial' hypercholesterolaemia is probably the commonest form of hypercholesterolaemia. The genetic basis is unclear, but there is failure to clear LDL cholesterol. Total cholesterol levels are in the range of 6.2-9.0 mmol/l and triglycerides are normal. It is associated with increased risk of coronary heart disease.
- Familial defective apolipoprotein B-100 is an autosomal dominant condition (prevalence = 1 in 600). Two mutations are described (arginine 3500 → glutamine; arginine 3531 → cysteine) in apo-B that impairs the binding of LDL to its receptor.

Combined Hyperlipidaemia

- Familial combined hyperlipidaemia (prevalence = 1 in 200 of the population). Coronary heart disease usually appears after the age of 60 years.
- Familial dysbetalipoproteinaemia, (prevalence = 1 in 3,000). It is also called remnant hyperlipidaemia, broad beta disease, or type III hyperlipidaemia. In these individuals remnant particles derived from the breakdown of chylomicrons and intermediate density lipoprotein (IDL) derived from VLDL are clear only very slowly, because they contain the Apo-E2 allele which has low affinity for its receptor. These patients present with palmar crease xanthoma, tuberous xanthoma on the elbows or knees, and premature coronary heart disease.

Secondary Hyperlipidaemia

The following list summarises the principle effect of various medical conditions on blood lipids (TG = triglyceride; TC = total cholesterol (or alternatively LDL cholesterol); HDL = HDL cholesterol; ↑ = increase; ↓ = decrease):

- Diabetes: ↑TG, ↑TC, ↓HDL
- Obesity: ↑TG
- Hypothyroidism: ↑TC, ↑TG
- Cholestasis: ↑TC
- Nephrotic syndrome: ↑TC
- Chronic renal failure: ↑TG, ↓HDL
- Alcoholism: ↑TG
- Drugs
  Beta blockers: ↑TG, ↓HDL
  Thiazides: ↑TG, ↑TC,
  Oestrogens: ↑TG, ↓TC, ↑HDL
  Androgens: ↓TG, ↑TC, ↓HDL
  Corticosteroid: ↑TG, ↑TC, ↑HDL
  Retinoic acid: ↑TG
  Phenytoin and phenobarbital: ↑HDL

Lipid Profiles

- Acute illness is associated with a fall in serum cholesterol and rise in triglyceride. It may take about 3 months before lipid levels return to baseline. However, lipid levels taken within 24 hours of an acute myocardial infarct are unaffected.
- Triglycerides rise postprandially, but total cholesterol and HDL cholesterol are unaffected.
- Triglyceride levels should be measured after a 9-12 hour fast.
- LDL cholesterol is calculated from fasting triglyceride, total cholesterol and HDL cholesterol using the Friedewald formula (all items are in mmol/l):

LDL cholesterol = (total cholesterol) − (HDL cholesterol) − (triglyceride ÷ 2.2)

Alternatively:

LDL cholesterol = (total cholesterol) − (HDL cholesterol) − (0.45 x triglyceride)

N.B. the Friedewald formula assumes that most of the triglyceride is contained in VLDL particles and that the ratio of triglyceride to cholesterol in VLDL is 2.2 to 1, which is not true if there is marked hypertriglyceridaemia or type III hyperlipidaemia. The Friedewald formula is, therefore, only valid if the triglyceride is less than 4.5 mmol/l. When the triglyceride is above 4.5 mmol/l, the LDL cholesterol can be directly measured using ultracentrifugation.

- Triglyceride levels of > 10 mmol/l will be associated with high cholesterol (8-15 mmol/l), because of the cholesterol contained in chylomicrons and VLDL rather than LDL particles. These patients should be first treated with triglyceride lowering medications.
- High total cholesterol can be due to high HDL cholesterol, especially in women. In these individuals the LDL cholesterol may be normal and would not require treatment.

Coronary Risk Prediction for Primary Prevention

The total cholesterol to HDL cholesterol ratio is used in the Joint British Societies Coronary Risk Prediction Chart, which gives the estimated risk of coronary heart disease for the purpose of *primary* prevention, and is found in the back pages of the British National Formulary. This Coronary Risk Prediction Chart is available as a free computer programme, which can be downloaded at the following internet websites:
www.bnf.org.uk
www.hyp.ac.uk/bhs/resources/guidelines.htm.

The Joint British Societies Coronary Risk Prediction Chart for Primary Prevention uses the following parameters:
- Total cholesterol to HDL cholesterol ratio
- Age (35–74 years)
- Sex of the individual
- Systolic BP
- Cigarette smoking
- Presence of diabetes

This Coronary Risk Prediction Chart is not usable in those with existing coronary heart disease or people with familial hypercholesterolaemia. Other exclusions apply.

The results are given as:
- CHD risk $\geq$ 30% over the next 10 years
- CHD risk 15-30% over the next 10 years
- CHD risk < 15% over the next 10 years

In the UK individuals with a very high CHD risk $\geq$ 30% over the next 10 years should receive cholesterol lowering treatment, as well as advice on blood pressure control, smoking, and lifestyle changes. If resources allow it is hoped that all individuals will be targeted for treatment if their CHD is above 15% over the next 10 years.

Recommended Targets for Cholesterol Treatment

In patients with coronary artery disease a 1% reduction in cholesterol level produces a 2% fall in cardiovascular mortality. For primary and secondary prevention of coronary artery disease, the desirable targets quoted in the British National Formulary (September 2002) are:
- total cholesterol concentration of < 5 mmol/l, *or*
  20-25% reduction in total cholesterol concentration,
  and use which ever is the lowest figure.
- LDL cholesterol of < 3 mmol/l, *or*
  30% reduction in LDL cholesterol,
  and use which ever is the lowest figure.

Triglycerides and Coronary Heart Disease

In the absence of co-existing hypercholesterolaemia, the treatment of hypertriglyceridaemia in someone without coronary heart disease (i.e. primary prevention) is controversial. In recent years the benefit of reducing triglycerides has been put forward for those with established coronary artery disease (i.e. secondary prevention of further cardiovascular events). The third report of the National Cholesterol Education Program (NCEP) in 2001 recommended a target triglyceride level of < 1.7 mmol/l. This is because hyper-triglyceridaemia is associated with the following harmful effects on lipid profiles:
- reduced HDL levels
- elevated LDL levels, especially small dense LDL particles which are more atherogenic

As noted previously it is not possible to calculate LDL-cholesterol using the Friedewald formula if the triglyceride is > 4.5 mmol/l. Triglyceride levels of > 10 mmol/l are associated with high cholesterol, which is contained in chylomicrons and VLDL rather than LDL particles. Secondary causes of hypertriglyceridaemia should be excluded and the minimum requirements are the following tests: fasting glucose, serum electrolytes, thyroid and liver function. These patients should be first treated with triglyceride lowering measures - which will also prevent acute pancreatitis - including diet, weight reduction, avoidance of alcohol, exercise, and fibrates or nicotinic acid. Only after triglyceride levels have been lowered to < 4.5 mmol/l should one's attention turn to LDL lowering therapy.

Treatment targets for hypertension and hyperlipidaemia in type 2 diabetes have been published by the UK's National Institute for Clinical Excellence (NICE) in October 2002. This document can be downloaded at the following website: *www.nice.org.uk.*

CASE 59

A 38-year-old man has large tonsils and the following fasting lipid profile:

Total cholesterol	4.6 mmol/l
LDL cholesterol	3.2 mmol/l
HDL cholesterol	0.7 mmol/l
Triglycerides	1.6 mmol/l

Question

What is this lipid disorder and describe its associated features?

Answer

This patient has Tangier's disease, which is associated with:

- Autosomal recessive inheritance
- Mutation in the ABC1 protein on chromosome 9
- ABC1 = ATP-binding cassette 1 transporter protein, which transports cholesterol out of cells to form apo-A1 particles. Failure to transport cholesterol out of cells leads to enlargement of organs.
- Heterozygotes have HDL levels of about half normal; HDL is absent in homozygotes.
- Enlarged yellow coloured tonsils that contain cholesterol
- Hepatosplenomegaly
- Neuropathy can present as pseudosyringomyelia, facial nerve palsy, or truncal neuropathy
- Corneal scarring from cholesterol deposits
- Premature coronary artery disease

Sitosterolaemia

Sitosterolaemia is an autosomal recessive disorder of plant sterol storage. It was first described in 1974 and to date there are only about 40 such cases worldwide. There is increased absorption of plant sterols such as sitosterol from the gastrointestinal tract and failure of the liver to eliminate sitosterol. There is also unexplained decreased cholesterol synthesis. Some laboratory assays cannot distinguish between cholesterol and plant sterols. Therefore, sitosterolaemia can be easily confused with hypercholesterolaemia. Mutations in two ATP-binding cassette (ABC) transporter proteins have been described: ABCG5 and ABCG8 on the small arm of chromosome 2. These two ABC transporters pump out plant sterols from the intestinal cells into the gut lumen and out of hepatic cells into the bile. Widespread deposition of sitosterol leads to premature coronary arterial disease, and xanthomas deposits in the tendons of the hands and Achilles tendon. Sterols also render red cell and platelet membranes more fragile and lead to haemolysis and thrombocytopenia. There is no response to Statins. The only treatments are dietary restriction in the intake of plant sterols and measures to reduce sterol absorption, such as ileal bypass surgery or use of bile acid binding resins.

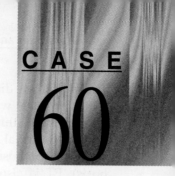
CASE 60

This is the blood count of a 78-year-old woman who had been admitted with a stroke.

Hb	12.6 g/dl
WBC	12.7 x 10⁹/l
Platelets	1,237 x 10⁹/l

Question

What are the diagnostic possibilities?

Answer

The most likely diagnosis is essential thrombocythaemia (ET), which presents with bleeding problems (especially gastrointestinal tract), thrombosis in arteries (TIAs, cerebral infarction, myocardial infarction, or peripheral ischaemia) and venous thrombosis (leg DVT, hepatic and splenic vein thrombosis). ET is also referred to as "primary thrombocytosis" or "primary thrombocythaemia". Treatments to reduce the platelet count include: hydroxycarbamide (hydroxyurea), platelet-pheresis, alpha interferon, radioactive phosphorus ^{32}P. Low dose aspirin is given for those who have predominantly thrombotic problems, such as digital ischaemia.

Elevations in platelet count, which are "reactive" or "secondary", occur in many conditions, including:

• Infection
• Chronic inflammation e.g. rheumatoid disease, inflammatory bowel disease
• Tissue trauma, surgery, and burns
• Haemorrhage
• Iron deficiency
• Post splenectomy
• Malignancy
• Chemotherapy

A one year prospective study of 777 patients with platelet counts greater than 500 x 10^9/l showed that 21% of the thrombocytosis cases were caused by infection, 19% involved rebound (after bleeding, iron deficiency, or cancer chemotherapy), 18% were a result of tissue damage, and 13% were due to chronic inflammation. Malignancy, splenectomy, and myeloproliferative disorders each accounted for fewer than 5% of cases. (Santhosh-Kumar CR, Yohannan MD, Higgy KE, al-Mashhadani SA. Thrombocytosis in adults: analysis of 777 patients. J Intern Med. 1991;229:493-495.)

Diagnostic Criteria for Essential Thrombocythaemia (ET)

ET is one of the myeloproliferative disorders (the others in this group are polycythaemia vera, myelofibrosis, and chronic myeloid leukaemia). An elevated platelet count also occurs in other myeloproliferative disorders, which must be excluded before the diagnosis of ET is sustainable. ET can transform into PV, myelofibrosis, or myeloid leukaemia. The Polycythaemia Vera Study Group has proposed the following criteria for essential thrombocythaemia:

- Platelet count > 600 x 10^9/l
- Hb < 13 g/dl or *normal* red cell mass (men < 36 ml/kg; women <32ml/kg)
- Stainable iron in the bone marrow
- No Philadelphia chromosome
- Absence of fibrosis in bone marrow
- No known cause of reactive thrombocytosis

Note: The above diagnostic criteria for ET remind clinicians to carefully exclude other myeloproliferative conditions *and* reactive causes of thrombocytosis. Splenomegaly may be present initially, but splenic infarction ultimately leads to splenic atrophy.

CASE 61

This asymptomatic 80-year-old has dipstick proteinuria.

Na	141 mmol/l
K	4.4 mmol/l
Urea	6.2 mmol/l
Creatinine	97 µmol/l
Albumin	35 g/l
Globulin	41 g/l
Bilirubin	5 µmol/l
ALP	81 U/l
ALT	13 U/l
Hb	13.3 g/dl
WBC	8.2 x 10⁹/l
Platelets	280 x 10⁹/l
ESR	48 mm/h
IgA	1.07 g/l (ref 0.7 – 4.0)
IgG	14.2 g/l (ref 5.4 – 16.5)
IgM	> 5.0 g/l (ref 0.5 –2)
Serum electrophoresis	IgM kappa monoclonal paraprotein (8 g/l)

Question
What is the most likely diagnosis?

Answer

The presence of paraproteinaemia is suggested by the raised serum globulin. This patient has monoclonal gammopathy of uncertain significance (MGUS).

Benign plasma cell proliferation is associated with the following clinical disorders:
* MGUS
* POEMS
* Primary systemic amyloidosis (i.e. Amyloid AL = light chain amyloidosis)

Malignant plasma cell proliferation is associated with:
* Myeloma
* Solitary plasmacytoma
* Waldenström's macroglobulinaemia. IgM monoclonal paraprotein is more likely to produce hyperviscosity syndrome and cold agglutinin mediated haemolytic anaemia, which are key features of Waldenström's macroglobulinaemia.

Monoclonal Gammopathy of Uncertain Significance (MGUS)

MGUS occurs in about 3% of people over the age of 70 years and has a good prognosis. The key features of MGUS are:
* Monoclonal paraproteinaemia is < 30 g/l
* There is no Bence-Jones proteinuria
  N.B. some diagnostic criteria for MGUS allow for a Bence-Jones proteinuria of < 1 g/day
* There are no osteolytic lesions
* There is no anaemia
* There is no hypercalcaemia
* There is no renal failure
* The concentration of plasma cells in the bone marrow is < 10%

Peripheral neuropathy may appear in 5-28% of patients with MGUS. IgM-MGUS is most often associated with neuropathy and has a predilection for large fibre involvement. Neuropathies associated with IgG-MGUS and IgA-MGUS respond better to plasma exchange than IgM-MGUS.

Patients with MGUS should have their paraproteinaemia checked periodically: 3-6 months from initial diagnosis and then annually if the quantity of paraproteinaemia is stable. However, 37% of patients with MGUS will show no disease progression over the next 10 years. Only 20% of patients with MGUS will develop a malignant plasma cell disorder (including myeloma, amyloidosis AL, and Waldenström's macroglobulinaemia) or lymphoma over a 10 year period.

POEMS or the Crowe-Fukase Syndrome

POEMS is a combination of:

- *Peripheral neuropathy* Segmental demyelination and axonal degeneration, with markedly reduced motor and sensory nerve conduction velocities, are due to complement mediated damage by antibodies to myelin-glycoproteins. The cerebrospinal fluid protein is high, but there is no increase in cell numbers.

- *Organomegaly* There is hepatomegaly (80% of patients), splenomegaly (25%), lymphadenopathy in the thorax or abdomen (60%)

- *Endocrinopathy* In women of child bearing age, amenorrhoea is common; in men the most common feature is gynaecomastia or impotence. Other associations are diabetes mellitus, Addison's disease, hypothyroidism, and hyperprolactinaemia.

- *Monoclonal gammopathy* There is an IgG monoclonal protein due to excess production of the lambda light chains. Lytic lesions can occur.

- *Skin changes* Hyperpigmentation, hirsutism, hyperhidrosis, and mucopolysaccharide containing plaques or papules.

CASE 62

This 40-year-old man has painful weakness in both shoulders and thighs. On examination, there was marked proximal weakness in the upper and lower limbs, but no other abnormal neurological signs. There was no evidence of joint disease or vascular disease. There was no response to prednisolone.

Hb	10.6 g/dl
WBC	6.4 x 10^9/l
Platelets	259 x 10^9/l
ESR	76 mm/h
Na	143 mmol/l
K	4.0 mmol/l
Urea	7.3 mmol/l
Creatinine	76 µmol/l
CK	110 U/l
Bilirubin	12 µmol/l
Albumin	36 g/l
Globulin	38 g/l
TSH	2.3 mU/l
ALP	357 U/l
AST	32 U/l
Corrected calcium	2.2 mmol/l
PO$_4$	0.5 mmol/l

Questions

1. What further investigations are needed?
2. What is the most likely diagnosis?

Answers

1. Further investigations should include:
   - Urinalysis for glycosuria, proteinuria, aminoaciduria, and acidic pH. These urinary abnormalities suggest Fanconi's syndrome.
   - Urinary phosphate excretion
   - X-rays of the chest and pelvis. Looser's zones are areas of defective mineralisation that occur in osteomalacia and are best seen in the ribs, scapulae and femurs
   - Bone biopsy to look for histological evidence of osteomalacia
   - PTH
   - Vitamin D
   - Prostate specific antigen and myeloma screening tests: Bence-Jones proteinuria, serum electrophoresis for monoclonal paraproteinaemia, bone marrow examination. Malignancy, including prostate and myeloma, can present as a painful proximal myopathy.

2. This patient has hypophosphataemic osteomalacia. The most important abnormality is a low serum phosphate with an elevated ALP. The treatment is oral phosphate and calcitriol, which improved all his symptoms. The lack of response to prednisolone makes the diagnosis of polymyagia rheumatica unlikely.

Causes of hypophosphataemic osteomalacia or rickets include:
- Hyperparathyroidism
- Malabsorption
- Vitamin D deficiency
- Renal tubular defects: Fanconi's syndrome
- X-linked vitamin D resistance
- Oncogenic osteomalacia, or "tumour rickets", is associated with mesenchymal tumours (such as haemangiopericytoma, haemangioma, non-ossifying fibroma), carcinoma of the prostate, oat cell carcinoma, myeloma, and chronic lymphatic leukaemia.
- Alcoholism
- Diabetes mellitus
- Respiratory alkalosis

CASE 63

A 64-year-old woman gave a 4 months history of anorexia, 6 kg weight loss, lower abdominal pain, and diarrhoea. The bowels were opened 4-6 times a day without rectal bleeding. In the previous 6 months she had several chest infections. Erosive rheumatoid arthritis was diagnosed 5 years ago and treated with NSAIDs and gold. She had pulmonary TB 20 years ago and duodenal ulcer 12 years ago. The current medications were loperamide and mefenamic acid. On examination, she was emaciated and afebrile. There was no finger clubbing, lymphadenopathy or organomegaly. The chest was clear.

Hb	10.5 g/dl
MCV	80 fl
WBC	12×10^9/l
ESR	48 mm/h
U&E	normal
Ca	2.6 mmol/l
PO_4	1.16 mmol/l
Bilirubin	8 μmol/l
ALP	300 U/l
AST	25 U/l
ALT	18 U/l
Albumin	39 g/l
Globulins	22 g/l
γ-GT	35 U/l

Questions
1. What is the most likely diagnosis?
2. Give two other causes for her diarrhoea.

Answers

1. Hypogammaglobuminaemia
2. The other two causes that have to be considered are: tuberculous enteritis and NSAID induced enteritis.

Hypogammaglobulinaemia

The humoral immune response by B-lymphocytes (B-cells) refers to the production of immunoglobulins with antibody properties that bind to foreign antigens on infectious agents and result in their elimination. The term gamma globulins refer to the electrophoretic mobility of these immunoglobulins. Each immunoglobulin molecule consists of two light and two heavy chains. The light chains are either lambda (λ) or kappa (k). There are 5 types of heavy chains, which form the basis of the 5 classes of immunoglobulins (IgG, IgA, IgM, IgD, IgE).

IgG has 4 subclasses. IgG1 reacts with protein antigens such as antitetanus and antidiphtheria antibodies. IgG2 and IgG4 react with polysaccharide antigens, e.g. antipneumococcal and haemophilus influenzae antibodies. IgG3 reacts with virus protein. IgA1, IgA2, and IgM are secreted by mucous membranes, and protect the respiratory and gastrointestinal tracts. IgA1 also appears in the blood. The biological function of IgD is unclear. IgE is involved in allergic responses and defences against nematode infections.

Abnormally low levels of gamma globulins or hypogammaglobulinaemia may be due to failure of production or excessive loss. As a result patients with hypogammaglobulinaemia are prone to recurrent infections, but there is also an increased risk of autoimmune disease and malignancy.

Causes of Hypogammaglobulinaemia

Most congenital causes of hypogammaglobulinaemia, such as Wiskott-Aldrich syndrome, present in childhood and lead to early death, and are not encountered by adult physicians. The following congenital disorders may appear in adults.

Congenital B-cell Disorders

- Common variable immunodeficiency. This is the most common cause of hypogammaglobulinaemia in adults and usually occurs in the second and third decade. There is failure of B-cell differentiation, which leads to very low levels of IgG. These patients present with recurrent chest infections (pneumococcus and Haemophilus influenzae), otitis media, sinusitis, diarrhoea (Giardia lamblia and Campylobacter species), severe viral infections (herpes zoster and herpes simplex), and fungal infections.

- Selective IgA deficiency. This can be autosomal recessive or dominant, or acquired. The majority of these patients are healthy, but a few individuals develop severe bronchiectasis often with cor pulmonale; associated conditions include coeliac disease, inflammatory bowel disease, rheumatoid disease, SLE and other autoimmune diseases. These patients develop IgE antibodies directed against the IgA contained in blood products. Subsequent blood transfusions can then lead to anaphylactic reactions. IgA deficiency can be acquired in some patients taking phenytoin, D-penicillamine, sulfasalazine, and hydroxychloro–quine.

- Selective IgM deficiency. This presents as life threatening infection with encapsulated bacteria, especially the pneumococcus and meningococcus.

- Immunoglobulin G subclass deficiency. IgG2 deficient patients develop recurrent infections from Haemophilus influenzae and pneumococcus, due to their inability to mount an effective antibody response to the polysaccharide antigens carried by these bacteria.

- Immunodeficiency with thymoma. Also known as Good's syndrome and the age of onset is around 40-70 years. Hypogammaglobulinaemia is seen in about 5% of patients with thymoma and does not resolve after thymectomy. Myasthenia gravis, pure red cell aplasia and agranulocytosis also occur, and improve after thymectomy.

- Immunoglobulin E hypogammaglobulinaemia. These patients are not at increased risk of infection, but have a high incidence of autoimmune disease and airflow obstruction.

- Bruton's disease, X-linked agammaglobulinaemia (XLA), affects only boys and is due to a tyrosine kinase genetic mutation (Bruton's tyrosine kinase gene, BTK) on the long arm of the X chromosome. As a result of this mutation B-cells fail to mature. IV immunoglobulin treatment allows patients with XLA to survival into adulthood.

- Bloom's syndrome (congenital telangiectatic erythema) is an autosomal recessive condition characterised by photosensitivity and deficiencies in both IgA and IgM. The photosensitivity improves with age, but malignancy (leukaemia, lymphoma, and gastrointestinal adenocarcinoma) is common in those who survive into the third decade. This syndrome is due to a mutation on chromosome 15, which codes for DNA helicase.

Combined B-cell and T-cell Disorder

- Adenosine deaminase deficiency leading to intracellular accumulation of deoxyadenosine triphosphate, which is toxic to B and T-lymphocytes, can appear in adult life as progressive failure of the immune system.

Acquired Disorders

- Severe malnutrition is the leading cause of acquired combined immunodeficiency worldwide.
- Catabolic states: nephrotic syndrome, protein-losing enteropathy, thyrotoxicosis.
- Immunosuppression therapy.
- Viral infection. Hypogammaglobulinaemia, especially low levels of IgG2, has been described with chronic Epstein-Barr virus infection.
- Lymphoproliferative malignancy: myeloma, chronic lymphocytic leukaemia, lymphomas.
- Severe ovarian hyperstimulation syndrome (OHSS). In severe OHSS, human chorionic gonadotrophin (hCG) leads to the production of multiple ovarian follicles and the release

of vascular endothelial growth factor (VEGF or vasculotropin) and interleukin-6 (IL-6). The increased capillary permeability from VEGF and IL-6 causes the formation of pleural effusion and ascites. Leakage of IgG and IgA into the peritoneal cavity results in hypogammaglobulinaemia.

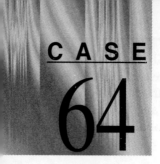

CASE 64

A 74-year-old woman was first admitted 2 years ago with hyponatraemia (Na 110 mmol/l) and hypokalaemia (K 3.2 mmol/l), which were thought to be side effects of her antihypertensive medication (bendroflumethiazide 5 mg od). The bendroflumethiazide was stopped and the hyponatraemia was successfully treated. However, sodium levels remained in the low normal range at many clinic visits and the blood pressure was difficult to control despite maximum doses of lisinopril, atenolol, and amlodipine. She was readmitted with breathlessness and swelling in both legs up to the groin and sacrum. The blood pressure was 200/110 mmHg and pulse 90 bpm. The jugular venous pressure was elevated to the right earlobe. There were no cardiac murmurs, but fine crackles could be heard in both lungs.

	Day 1 (most recent admission)	Day 5 (after IV furosemide)
Na	114 mmol/l	133 mmol/l
K	4.2 mmol/l	4.2 mmol/l
Urea	4.0 mmol/l	4.3 mmol/l
Creatinine	61 µmol/l	84 µmol/l
Albumin	40 g/l	
Globulin	31 g/l	
Bilirubin	10 µmol/l	
ALP	163 U/l	
ALT	30 U/l	
TSH	4.1 mU/l	
Serum osmolality	241 mosmol/kg	
Urine osmolality	477 mosmol/kg	
Urinalysis	normal	
CXR	cardiomegaly	
ECG	left ventricular hypertrophy	

Question
What is the cause of this patient's hyponatraemia?

Answer

This patient has severe dilutional hyponatraemia. This was due to the ingestion of liquorice confectionery, which encouraged water retention in relative excess of sodium retention. Other effects of liquorice include hypertension and hypokalaemia. In this patient the absence of hypokalaemia may be due to lisinopril. She was advised to eschew liquorice sweets and since then her hypertension has been much easier to control and there has been no recurrence of the fluid retention.

Liquorice Toxicity

Liquorice is an extract from the root of *Glycyrrhiza glabra* and is used as a flavouring agent in sweets and breath fresheners. Liquorice contains glycyrrhizic acid (GZA), which is metabolised to 18 β-glycyrrhetinic acid (GRA). Both GZA and GRA inhibit the enzyme 11 β-hydroxysteroid dehydrogenase (11β-HSD) and leads to a hypermineralocorticoid syndrome or "pseudo-primary hyperaldosteronism".

- Cortisol and aldosterone have the same affinity for the mineralocorticoid receptor in the distal renal tubule. However, 11β-HSD protects mineralocorticoid receptors from the stimulatory effects of cortisol by converting it to inactive corticosterone.
- Inhibition of 11β-HSD by GZA in liquorice produces excess cortisol and reduces corticosterone.
- Excess cortisol binds to mineralocorticoid receptors in the kidneys to produce:
  a. sodium and water retention (hypertension and oedema)
  b. potassium excretion (hypokalaemic muscle weakness/ rhabdomyolysis/arrhythmias)
  c. hydrogen ion excretion (metabolic alkalosis)

Therefore, typical changes in liquorice toxicity are:
- Plasma renin activity and aldosterone are low
- Urine aldosterone is low
- Urine free cortisol is high
- Urine corticosterone is low
- Urine cortisol-corticosterone metabolite ratio is high

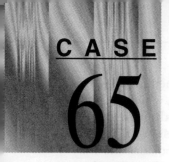

C A S E

65

CASE 65

A 72-year-old woman was admitted with sudden onset severe epigastric pain, which radiated into the back, and vomiting. Two years ago she had undergone a laparoscopic cholecystectomy. On examination, she was markedly obese (BMI = 37), the pulse was 90 bpm, BP 137/82 mmHg, temperature 36.7° Celsius. There was some tenderness in the upper abdomen, but no masses were present and the bowel sounds were normal. The chest and heart were unremarkable. The pain disappeared after 24 hours and did not recur. The ECG, chest and abdominal X-rays were normal.

Hb	14.3 g/dl
WBC	$7.3 \times 10^9/l$
Platelets	$220 \times 10^9/l$
MCV	89.2 fl
CRP	22 mg/l
Prothrombin time	9.8 seconds
INR	0.9
Na	131 mmol/l
K	3.8 mmol/l
Urea	4 mmol/l
Creatinine	77 µmol/l
Glucose	8.8 mmol/l
Albumin	44 g/l
Globulin	36 g/l
Bilirubin	44 µmol/l
ALP	379 U/l
γ-GT	1044 U/l
ALT	773 U/l
AST	698 U/l
Corrected calcium	2.25 mmol/l
Amylase	33 U/l

Questions

1. What are the next steps in investigations?
2. What is the most likely diagnosis?

Answers

In most hospitals the laboratory results for "liver function tests" will include one or both aminotransaminases (also called aminotransferases: ALT and AST) and alkaline phosphatase. ALT is found predominantly in the liver, but AST occurs in various tissues, including the heart, skeletal muscle, kidney, brain and liver. Elevation in the aminotransaminases is often called a 'hepatitic' or 'hepatocellular' pattern, because the cause is usually some form of hepatocellular damage. In contrast, elevation in the alkaline phosphatase indicates cholestasis and is referred to as a 'cholestatic' pattern. A mixed pattern, i.e. elevation in both aminotransferase and alkaline phosphatase, is more commonly encountered especially in cardiac failure, fatty liver, and some types of drug induced reactions.

Conditions Associated with a Predominantly Elevated ALT or AST

- Acute hepatitis: viral, alcohol, or drugs (e.g. NSAIDs, statins, isoniazid, allopurinol)
- Chronic hepatitis and cirrhosis: viral, autoimmune, or metabolic (e.g. haemochromatosis, Wilson's disease, alpha$_1$ antitrypsin deficiency)
- Fatty liver (hepatic steatosis) and non-alcoholic steatohepatitis (NASH): occurs in obesity, hyperlipidaemia, and diabetes
- Muscle injury or inflammation: myocardial infarction, trauma, surgery, myositis
- Acute biliary obstruction: AST and ALT reach a peak at 48 hours and levels may be > 300 U/l, but then decline rapidly.
- In alcoholic hepatitis the aminotransferases are only modestly elevated (< 300 U/l) and the ratio of AST/ALT is > 2.0. Look also for macrocytosis and elevated GT (γ-GT), which is induced by alcohol.
- Much higher aminotransferase levels (> 300 U/l) occur in viral hepatitis and the AST/ALT ratio is typically < 1.0.
- Very high aminotransferases (> 2-3,000 U/l) occur in drug-induced liver necrosis, including paracetamol poisoning, severe viral hepatitis, and sepsis.

Conditions Associated with a Predominantly Elevated Alkaline Phosphatase

These include hepatobiliary disease, bony pathology, and physiological conditions:

- Intrahepatic cholestasis: primary biliary cirrhosis, sclerosing cholangitis, drug induced liver disease (e.g. neuroleptics, flucloxacillin, augmentin, erythromycin, testosterone), malignancy (hepatoma and secondary deposits), infiltrations (amyloidosis, granulomas), cardiac failure, sepsis.
- Extrahepatic cholestasis: gall stones, carcinoma of pancreas, benign or malignant biliary strictures.
- Elevations in both alkaline phosphatase *and* γ-GT indicate hepatobiliary disease.
- Elevation in alkaline phosphatase *without* elevation in γ-GT suggests bone disease, such as fracture, bony metastases, and Paget's disease.
- Isolated elevation in γ-GT is most often due to enzyme induction, including alcohol and drugs (e.g. phenytoin).
- Physiological conditions that produce mild elevations (< 3 times the upper limit of normal) in alkaline phosphatase are adolescence (due to growing bones) and pregnancy (due to placenta).

Other LFT tests

Bilirubin

- Bilirubin is derived mainly from red cell breakdown
- Bilirubin is conjugated in the liver and excreted in the bile
- Elevated unconjugated (indirect) bilirubin occurs in haemolysis, Gilbert's syndrome and Crigler-Najjar syndrome.
- Elevated conjugated (direct) bilirubin occurs in hepatobiliary disease and congenital conjugated hyperbilirubinaemia (Dubin-Johnson and Rotor syndromes)

Albumin and Globulin

- Hypoalbuminaemia suggests chronic liver disease, but low levels also occur in many disorders: poor diet, chronic illness, nephrotic syndrome, protein losing enteropathy, etc.
- Raised globulins: elevated IgG in autoimmune chronic hepatitis; elevated IgM in primary biliary cirrhosis; elevated IgA in alcoholic liver disease.

Clotting Factors

- The liver synthesises clotting factors II, VII, IX, X (which are vitamin K dependent) and factor V (which is not vitamin K dependent).
- Factor V levels may help to distinguish between liver disease from vitamin K deficiency.
- Prothrombin time is widely used to provide information on the severity and prognosis of liver disease.

Further Investigations in this Patient

In this patient the sudden onset of abdominal pain with disturbed LFTs should suggest gallstones, which can recur after a cholecystectomy. In the early stages of biliary obstruction, the rise in serum transaminases may exceed that of ALP. After a few days these aminotransaminases return to normal, but if the obstruction persists the blood test will revert to 'cholestatic' pattern and show a predominant rise in alkaline phosphatase. If the transaminases remain high, one should consider one of the causes of a 'hepatitic' pattern. So further investigations in this patient should include:

- Review medication history and alcohol intake
- Repeat liver function tests
- Autoimmune serology (antismooth and antimitochondrial antibody)
- Viral hepatitis serology (hepatitis A, B, C)
- Abdominal ultrasound
- ERCP if there is ultrasound evidence of biliary obstruction

Repeat LFTs at 18 days after admission

Albumin	39 g/l
Globulin	24 g/l
Bilirubin	16 µmol/l
ALT	123 U/l
ALP	170 U/l
ANA	less than 1 in 40
Antimitochondrial antibody	negative
Antismooth muscle antibody	negative
Hepatitis A IgM antibody	negative
Hepatitis B surface antigen	negative

Hepatitis B core antibody   negative
Hepatitis C antibody   negative
Liver ultrasound   fatty liver only

Non-Alcoholic Fatty Liver Disease (NAFLD)

The term non-alcoholic fatty liver disease (NAFLD) is used to describe a spectrum of liver disorders that are not due to alcohol, although the histology is similar to alcoholic hepatitis, including the presence of 'Mallory bodies'. NAFLD includes:

- Hepatic steatosis (fatty liver)
- Hepatic steatosis with non-specific inflammation
- Non-alcoholic steatohepatitis (NASH) in which there is steatosis plus hepatocyte ballooning degeneration, fibrosis, and neutrophilic inflammation, with or without Mallory bodies.

Prevalence of NAFLD

- Post mortem studies on individuals who die from accidents show a prevalence rate of 20% for hepatic steatosis and 3% for NASH.
- The prevalence of both hepatic steatosis and NASH is much greater among with individuals with insulin resistance syndrome, especially those with obesity and type 2 diabetes mellitus.

Aetiology of NAFLD

In addition to obesity and type 2 diabetes, NAFLD is associated with:

- Drugs (corticosteroids, tamoxifen, estrogen, amiodarone, calcium antagonists)
- Surgery (gastric surgery for obesity, extensive small bowel resection, jejuno-ileal bypass)
- Partial lipodystrophy
- Total parenteral nutrition with glucose

Pathophysiology of NAFLD

- Insulin resistance with failure to suppress peripheral lipolysis results in excess levels of circulating fatty acids.
- Hepatic uptake of fatty acid leads to increased triglyceride synthesis and fatty change in the liver.

- Fatty acid oxidation produces free radicals (which cause hepatocyte injury) and stimulates cytokine release (which attract neutrophils and stimulate hepatic fibrosis).

Diagnosis of NAFLD

- Patients with NAFLD are usually asymptomatic and deranged liver function tests and hepatomegaly are incidental findings during the investigation of other conditions. Similarly fatty liver may be a chance finding when ultrasound or CT scan is performed for other clinical reasons.
- Transaminase (AST and ALT) levels are elevated 2-3 times above the normal range. Higher levels are unusual. In about half of patients, γ-GT and ALP are also elevated 2-3 times. Serum bilirubin and albumin are normal, unless the condition has advanced to cirrhosis.
- Other causes of deranged LFT need to be excluded, especially alcohol excess, iron overload, and viral hepatitis.
- Accurate diagnosis of NAFLD requires liver biopsy, which also excludes other causes of disturbed liver function. Liver histology provides prognostic information on NAFLD and helps in deciding on its treatment options. Note: many of these pharmacological treatments (described below) are themselves potentially hepatotoxic.

Treatment of NAFLD

- Weight reduction has been shown to reduce serum transaminases levels and improve liver histology.
- Treatment of diabetes e.g. metformin may improve liver function tests and histology. Troglitazone has been shown to reduce liver enzyme levels in NAFLD, but is no longer available due to reports of liver toxicity.
- Treatment of hyperlipidaemia. Gemfibrozil, but not clofibrate, will reduce triglyceride levels and serum transaminases.
- Antioxidants such as acetylcysteine and vitamin E show promising effects on liver function, but require further evaluation.
- Ursodeoxycholic acid improves liver function tests and histology.

Prognosis of NAFLD

- Hepatic steatosis without fibrosis or inflammation has a relatively benign prognosis.
- Approximately 25% of patients with NASH will progress to cirrhosis over a 10 year period. It is these patients who may be offered pharmacological treatment.

Reference: McCullough AJ. Update on non-alcoholic fatty liver disease. J Clin Gastroenterol 2002;34(3):255-262.

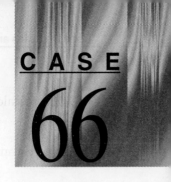

C A S E
66

CASE 66

A 71-year-old woman had fallen accidentally and struck her head. There was no loss of consciousness. Her memory had been poor during the last 3 years and her husband had taken over the housework, cooking and shopping. She was on no regular medications. There was no history of alcohol abuse. She was more confused after the fall, became doubly incontinent, wandered aimlessly around the house, and attempted to escape into the street at night. A hospital admission was quickly arranged by her General Practitioner. The physical examination was difficult as she was aggressive, swore profusely, and did not co-operate. The pulse was 72 bpm, BP 137/85 mmHg, and temperature 36.4° Celsius. There was bruising around both eyes, but no obvious focal neurological deficits. The chest, heart and abdomen were unremarkable. She was sedated with IV diazepam and the following investigations performed:

Na	135 mmol/l
K	4.2 mmol/l
Urea	4.4 mmol/l
Creatinine	99 µmol/l
Hb	13.7 x 10^9/l
WBC	9.3 x 10^9/l
Platelets	350 x 10^9/l
MCV	94 fl
TSH	1.81 mU/l
Free T4	18.5 pmol/l
Prolactin	237 mU/l (ref < 600)
LH	41.3 U/l
FSH	76.0 U/l
Bilirubin	12 µmol/l
Albumin	44 g/l
Globulin	32 g/l

ALP	95 U/l
ALT	22 U/l
Corrected calcium	normal
CXR	normal
ECG	normal
CT brain scan	cerebral atrophy, 1 cm pituitary tumour

Questions

1. Give three diagnoses.
2. What are the next steps in investigation?

Answers
1. Acute confusional state
2. Dementia
3. Pituitary incidentaloma

It is likely that this elderly woman has had a dementing process for the last 3 years, possibly Alzheimer's disease. The head injury has precipitated an acute confusional state and a subdural haematoma needed to be excluded by an urgent CT brain scan. However, acute confusion can have many other causes. The pituitary tumour has obviously nothing to do with her presenting illness. It is, therefore, referred to as an "incidentaloma", implying that it is found completely by chance in someone who has had a CT brain scan for other reasons.

Acute Confusional State
(synonyms: acute brain failure, delirium, toxic confusion)
An acute confusion state is a transient, global disorder of cognition and attention, with reduced consciousness, abnormally increased or reduced psychomotor activity and a disturbed sleep-wake cycle.

Risk Factors for Acute Confusion
- Very elderly or young
- Poor sight and hearing
- Underlying chronic brain failure (e.g. Alzheimer's and multi-infarct brain disease)
- Concurrent medications (e.g. antidepressants, L-dopa) and alcohol
- Change in environment
- Physical illness (especially infections, dehydration, and biochemical disturbance)

Key Diagnostic Features
1. Disordered thinking, altered perception and impaired memory:
   - drowsiness
   - disorientation
   - poor attention span, easily distracted

- delusions, hallucinations, paranoia
- restlessness, bewilderment
- abnormal sleep-wake cycle (especially nocturnal confusion 'Sundowners')
- poor memory and amnesia

2. Abrupt onset, variability in the severity of confusion, with lucid intervals.

Aide-Mémoire of Causes

1. Intracranial:
   - infarction (or haemorrhagic stroke, subdural haema toma)
   - infection (meningitis, encephalitis)
   - injuries to head
   - iatrogenic (drugs)
2. Extracranial:
   - infection (especially chest or urine)
   - insults of a metabolic nature (salt and water imbalance, hypoglycaemia, hyperglycaemia, hypoxia, alcohol, thiamine deficiency)

Treatment of Acute Confusional State

1. Reassure patient, relatives and medical staff
2. Treat any underlying cause.
3. Review medication list.
4. Careful fluid and electrolyte balance.
5. Treat agitation (haloperidol 0.5 mg bd orally, risperidone 0.5 mg od or bd orally, or IM/IV Diazepam, especially if alcohol withdrawal is suspected).

Reference: Lipowski ZJ. Delirium in the elderly patient. NEJM 1989:320:578-582.

Pituitary Incidentaloma

Post mortem studies have suggested that 13% of elderly people dying from other causes will harbour a pituitary tumour. During life the incidental finding of pituitary tumour is due to CT or MRI scan for other indications and these patients will be asymptomatic. The course of action for these incidentalomas include:

1. Assessment of visual fields to exclude compression of the optic chiasma.
2. Exclude hormonal hypersecretion:
   a. Exclude Cushing's disease by the overnight dexamethasone suppression test: give 1mg of dexamethasone at midnight and measure the 9 am cortisol. A normal response is suppression of the 9 am serum cortisol to < 50 nmol/l. Alternatively, measure the urinary free cortisol in a 24 hour urine sample.
   b. Exclude acromegaly. The diagnosis of acromegaly relies on demonstrating elevated GH levels (> 10 mU/l) during a 75 gram glucose tolerance test (GTT). Suppression of GH values to less than 2 mU/l at some point during the 2 hour GTT excludes the diagnosis of acromegaly. The production of Somatomedin-C or Insulin like Growth Factor 1 (IGF-1) by the liver is stimulated by GH. IGF-1 circulates bound to IGF binding protein 3. Levels of both IGF-1 and IGF binding protein 3 are elevated in acromegaly, allowing both tests to be used for diagnosis and assessing treatment response.
   c. Exclude hyperprolactinaemia. Venepuncture and many drugs (e.g. anti-psychotic drugs and anti-emetics) can cause a modest rise in prolactin levels. Prolactin levels of > 3,000 mU/l generally suggest prolactinoma.
   d. TSH-omas (or thyrotropinomas) i.e. TSH secreting pituitary tumours are exceedingly rare and suggested by an unsuppressed TSH and elevated T4.
3. Exclude hypopituitarism i.e. demonstrate deficiencies in anterior pituitary hormones (ACTH, TSH, LH, FSH, GH, prolactin) and posterior pituitary hormone (mainly ADH) secretion. A water deprivation test is needed to assess ADH secretion. Tests of anterior pituitary function includes:
   a. Prolactin
   b. FSH, LH, testosterone or estradiol
   c. TSH, free T4 and free T3
   d. 9 am cortisol
   e. Short Synacthen Test
   f. Insulin Tolerance Test (ITT)
   g. Glucagon Stimulation Test

Prolactin deficiency is very rare. Hyperprolactinaemia is much commoner, because damage to the pituitary stalk cuts off the inhibitory effect of dopamine from the hypothalamus on pituitary prolactin release. In postmenopausal women the gonadotrophin levels are very high (LH and FSH are typically > 40 U/l), so the finding of undetectable levels of LH and FSH is a strong pointer towards the diagnosis of hypopituitarism in this age group. In men a low serum testosterone with low FSH and LH should also suggest hypopituitarism. Low serum TSH, low free T4 and low free T3 may be difficult to distinguish form Sick Euthyroid Syndrome. Secretion of ACTH and cortisol are pulsatile with marked diurnal variation, with the highest values at 9am. An *abnormal* Short Synacthen Test in hypopituitarism is due to adrenal atrophy resulting from ACTH deficiency. However, a *normal* Short Synacthen Test does not completely rule out ACTH deficiency or hypopituitarism.

In the ITT hypoglycaemia (plasma glucose < 2.5 mmol/l) is produced by an IV insulin infusion. The dose of IV insulin is 0.15U per kg body weight, but a smaller dose is used in patients known to have hypoadrenalism or hypothyroidism. Insulin induced hypoglycaemia triggers the release of ACTH, Cortisol and GH. Glucagon (1 mg subcutaneously) produces an initial rise in blood glucose, which then stimulates endogenous insulin release and results in a hypoglycaemic effect. The ITT and Glucagon Test are usually combined with the TRH test and LH/FSH releasing hormone (Gonadotrophin releasing hormone, GnRH) test. TRH causes spasm of smooth muscle and is, therefore, unsafe in pregnant women and subjects with angina and asthma. Insulin induced hypoglycaemia is dangerous in elderly subjects, in whom the Glucagon Test may be safer.

4. Follow up MRI or CT scans of incidentaloma to detect tumour enlargement. Tumours of less than 1 cm can be re-scanned annually, but larger tumours will require more frequent scans.

CASE 67

A 46-year-old woman is known to have hepatitis B related liver disease. She now presented with increasing jaundice, ascites, and tender hepatomegaly.

Hb	9.1 g/dl
WBC	3.2 x 10⁹/l
Neutrophils	1.8 x 10⁹/l
Lymphocytes	1.0 x 10⁹/l
Monocytes	0.3 x 10⁹/l
Platelets	16 x 10⁹/l
MCV	104.8 fl
ESR	44 mm/h
Na	138 mmol/l
K	3.1 mmol/l
Urea	1.6 mmol/l
Creatinine	72 µmol/l
Glucose	5.8 mmol/l
Albumin	23 g/l
Globulin	42 g/l
Bilirubin	84 µmol/l
ALP	204 U/l
ALT	78 U/l
INR	1.8

Questions
1. Why is there a neutropenia and thrombocytopenia?
2. What may have caused the deterioration in liver function?

Answers

1. Neutropenia and thrombocytopenia may be due to:
   - hypersplenism
   - hepatitis B related bone marrow suppression
2. Deterioration in liver function may be due to:
   - superinfection with another hepatitis virus
   - development of hepatoma
   - side effect of alcohol or drugs

Other chronic complications from hepatotropic viruses are summarised in the table on the "viral hepatitis alphabet".

The Viral Hepatitis Alphabet

Viral hepatitis refers to an acute infection of the liver by a number of hepatotropic viruses, which may be followed by long term complications. It is customary to label viral hepatitis under the following letters of the alphabet: A, B, C, D, E, G. This nomenclature ignores the hepatitis infrequently produced by other viral pathogens, such as adenovirus, cytomegalovirus, Epstein-Barr virus, and herpes simplex virus.

Virus type	Nucleic acid structure	Main route of transmission	Long term complications
HAV	RNA Picornavirus	Faeco-oral	Acute infection only; no chronic disease.
HBV	DNA Hepadnavirus	Parenteral Sexual Perinatal	90-95% of adults with acute infections recover fully. 5-10% become chronic carriers 70-90% of chronic carriers are healthy but infectious. 10-30% of chronic carriers develop chronic hepatitis. 20% of chronic carriers (= 1% of all infected adults) will eventually develop cirrhosis or hepatoma.
HCV	RNA Flavirus	Parenteral Sexual	15% of adults with acute infection recover completely. The remaining 85% are at risk of developing chronic disease, including chronic hepatitis, cirrhosis and hepatoma.

Contd...

Contd...

Virus type	Nucleic acid structure	Main route of transmission	Long term complications
			20% of patients with chronic HCV eventually develop cirrhosis after a lapse of 10-20 years.
HDV	RNA 'delta virus'	Parenteral Sexual	HDV uses the HBsAg as its envelope protein and co-infection with HBV is needed to produce severe liver disease.
		Perinatal	Long term complications of HDV& HBV co-infection are the same as those described for pure HBV infection, but progression to cirrhosis is more rapid.
HEV	RNA Calcivirus	Faeco-oral	Acute infection only; no chronic disease. High mortality in pregnancy (>10%).
HGV	RNA Flavivirus	Parenteral Perinatal	HGV is common in patients on haemodialysis, renal transplant recipients, and haemophiliacs. No chronic complications from HGV infection. HGV co-infection with HBV or HCV is also frequent.
TTV	DNA	Parenteral Perinatal	Co-infection with HAV, HBV, HCV, or HEV is described. Mother to child transmission occurs. Chronic infection is common and not associated with liver disease.

Historical Notes:
Hepatitis F was first suggested in 1994 but remains unconfirmed.
Hepatitis G was identified by 2 independent groups in 1995-6. It is also called GB virus C.
Transfusion Transmissable Virus (TTV) was identified in 1977.
SEN-V (a DNA virus) was described in 2001 as a possible new hepatotropic virus.

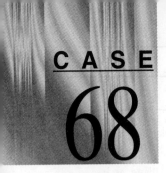

CASE 68

A 46-year-old woman presented with 6 months history of increasing breathlessness and chest pain precipitated by exercise. There was no response to nitrates, beta-blockers or calcium antagonists. About 3 months ago she develop bilateral ankle oedema and was started on furosemide. She was a non-smoker and teetotal. There was no family history of premature coronary artery disease and hypertension. For the past one year, she had been taking fenfluramine for weight reduction. Type 2 diabetes mellitus had been diagnosed for the past three years and treated by diet only.

Hb	16.2 g/dl
Haematocrit	51.2 l/l
MCV	103 fl
WBC	$7.5 \times 10^9/l$
Platelets	$189 \times 10^9/l$
Na	138 mmol/l
K	4.8 mmol/l
Urea	6.2 mmol/l
Creatinine	135 µmol/l
Bilirubin	32 µmol/l
AST	24 U/l
ALT	20 U/l
Albumin	40 g/l
Globulin	29 g/l
ECG	normal
CXR	normal

Questions
1. What other investigations are required?
2. What is the most likely diagnosis?

Answers

1. The following investigations would be useful:
   - Arterial blood gases
   - Lung function tests
   - Echocardiography
   - Right heart catheterisation
   - Pulmonary angiography
2. Fenfluramine induced pulmonary hypertension.

Causes of Pulmonary Hypertension

1. Primary Pulmonary Hypertension (PPH)
   - Idiopathic
   Primary pulmonary hypertension affects young women and people in the 5th-6th decade. There is no apparent cause. The incidence is two cases per million each year. It is traditional to include the two following clinical entities within the umbrella term of 'primary pulmonary hypertension'—
     - Drug induced: fenfluramine, cocaine, amfetamine, aminoplex
     - Familial: this is associated with a genetic defect on the long arm of chromosome 2
2. Secondary Pulmonary Hypertension
   - Chronic hypoxic lung disease
   - Chronic left heart failure
   - Chronic thromboembolic disease
   - Congenital cyanotic heart disease
   - Systemic lupus erythematosus
   - Systemic sclerosis
   - Sarcoidosis
   - Obesity
   - HIV infection
   - Chronic liver disease

Clinical Features

- Breathlessness
- Chest pain
- Syncope
- Fatigue

- Loud pulmonary component of the second heart sound, which is either fixed or paradoxically split.
- Tricuspid regurgitation
- Right ventricular hypertrophy (i.e. parasternal heave)
- Signs of right heart failure including raised jugular venous pressure and pulsatile liver.

Investigations

- Chest X-ray may show enlarged pulmonary arteries, the hyperinflated lungs of Chronic Obstructive Pulmonary Disease, interstitial lung disease, but may also be normal
- ECG may show P pulmonale (tall P waves) and right ventricular hypertrophy (tall R wave in V1 with ST depression and T wave inversion).
- Arterial blood gases or oximetry to assess suitability for long term oxygen therapy (LTOT)
- Lung function test to identify obstructive and restrictive lung disease
- High resolution chest CT and ventilation/perfusion lung scans to exclude interstitial lung disease and pulmonary thromboembolism.
- Echocardiography with Doppler to assess cardiac function, estimate pulmonary arterial pressure and identify congenital heart lesions.
- Cardiac catheterisation to assess haemodynamic response to vasodilators.
- Pulmonary angiography to exclude thromboembolic disease

Treatment Options in PPH

- Treatment of right heart failure (diuretics and digoxin)
- Anticoagulation
- Calcium channel blockers. Nifedipine and diltiazem.
- Prostacyclin analogues can be given IV, nebulised, or taken orally. Epoprostenol (Flolan) is given continuously through a central venous catheter using a battery-driven infusion pump.
- Endothelin receptor antagonist. Bosentan is an orally administered endothelin-1 receptor antagonist that reduces

pulmonary arterial resistance, pulmonary arterial pressure and right atrial pressure
- Inhaled nitric oxide
- Balloon atrial septostomy
- Heart and lung transplantation

Treating other types of Pulmonary Hypertension
- LTOT for patients with chronic hypoxic lung disease and cyanotic heart disease
- Anticoagulation and IVC filter (Greenfield catheter) to prevent further pulmonary embolism.
- Pulmonary embolectomy surgery carries a high risk for death or disability, and is rarely undertaken.

Prognosis of PPH

The following features suggest poor prognosis:
- NYHA grade 3 or 4
- Less than 500 metre walking distance over a 12 minute period.
- Cardiac index < 2 litres/min/m²
- Right atrial pressure > 20 mmHg
- Pulmonary arterial pressure > 85 mmHg

Good prognostic signs are:
- A 20% rise in cardiac output with IV prostacyclin
- A 30% fall in mean pulmonary arterial pressure with nitric oxide
- These two groups of patients may also benefit from oral calcium channel blockers.

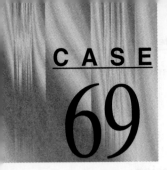

C A S E
69

CASE 69

An 85-year-old man presented to the A&E department with severe epigastric pain, which came on suddenly three hours earlier. This pain radiated across the upper abdomen and through to the back. It was associated with vomiting and mild breathlessness. Past medical history included hypertension. He drank moderate amounts of alcohol, but did not smoke cigarettes. On examination, the temperature was 36.7°Celsius, pulse 100 bpm regular, BP 161/88 mmHg (right arm) and 174/78 mmHg (left arm). The respiratory rate was 32 per minute and oxygen saturation 93% on room air. The JVP was 1 cm above the sternal angle. The cardiac apex was not displaced, the trachea was central in position, and the breath sounds were vesicular in character. There was epigastric tenderness, but no rigidity. He was alert with no focal neurological deficit.

Hb	12.2 g/dl
WBC	$3.4 \times 10^9/l$
Platelet	$243 \times 10^9/l$
MCV	87.4 fl
MCH	28.7 pg
Na	135 mmol/l
K	3.5 mmol/l
Urea	12.2 mmol/l
Creatinine	134 µmol/l
Glucose	13.2 mmol/l
Amylase	134 U/l
ECG	sinus tachycardia and left axis deviation
	T wave inversion in the left anterolateral chest leads
CXR	Right mid zone consolidation and raised left hemidiaphragm.

The provisional diagnosis was a lower respiratory tract infection and the differential diagnoses were acute cholecystitis and acute pancreatitis. Antibiotic treatment was commenced. Eight hours after attending hospital he became breathless at rest. Re-examination showed massive swelling of the neck consistent with surgical emphysema. A repeat chest X-ray confirmed subcutaneous emphysema with mediastinal emphysema, but there was no pneumothorax. He was hypoxic and the blood gases on air were as follows:

pH	7.4
PCO_2	4.7 kPa
PO_2	7.1 kPa
HCO_3	22 mmol/l
Base excess	- 4 mmol/l

The patient was reviewed by the medical senior registrar who made the correct clinical diagnosis.

Question
What was the diagnosis?

Answer

Boerhaave's syndrome; spontaneous rupture of the oesophagus.

Boerhaave's Syndrome

Hermann Boerhaave, a Dutch physician, is credited with the first description of this syndrome that now bears his name. A common habit in the 18th century was to induce vomiting so that more food can be eaten. The first reported patient with Boerhave's syndrome was the Grand Admiral of Netherlands, who at age of 50 years induced vomiting for 18 hours, which resulted in an oesophageal rupture. At postmortem, the left pleural cavity was found to contain olive oil and roasted duck. There was also a transverse tear at the lower end of the oesophagus.

Vomiting while the cricopharyngeus is closed causes a sudden rise in intra-oesophageal pressure and leads to oesophageal rupture. The oesophageal tear is usually longitudinal, 2-3 cm long, and located at the lower end of the oesophagus on the left side (75-90% of cases). This is the weakest point of the oesophagus as it is not supported by other organs, the muscular layer is also thin with segmental defects in the circular layer, and is the point of entry of vessels and nerves. The lower oesophagus is angulated anteriorly at the left diaphragmatic crux. The rupture is bilateral in 5-10% of cases and it is rare for a rupture to occur only at the right side. Leakage of gastric contents (acid, enzymes, food and bacteria) across the oesophageal tear causes mediastinitis, which may present as:

1. Shock
2. Cardio-respiratory failure
3. Fluid losses
4. Suppuration in the mediastinum and pleural cavity

The classical clinical presentation of Boerhaave's syndrome includes overindulgence in food or drink followed by:

- Severe pain in the chest or abdomen. The chest pain is usually left sided, pleuritic in nature, and may radiate through to the back. The pain usually does not respond to narcotics.

- Breathlessness due to pain, pneumothorax or hydropneumothorax
- Mediastinal or subcutaneous emphysema is seen in 28 to 66% of patients
- Cardiovascular collapse with hypotension
- Chest X-ray showing pneumothorax or hydropneumothorax

However, unusual clinical features include:
- Extreme swelling of the face and neck
- Polydipsia
- Pericarditis
- Pneumoperitoneum
- Pneumopericardium
- Proptosis
- Change of voice
- Ruptured diaphragm
- Low pleural fluid amylase

Diagnosis of Boerhaave's Syndrome

The diagnosis is commonly missed with < 35% of the patients being diagnosed ante-mortem, because of:
- Incomplete clinical history
- Diagnostic difficulty if there was no history of vomiting
- Signs of surgical emphysema may be easily missed, especially if it is limited in distribution
- Chest X-ray may not have been requested if the patient presented with abdominal pain
- Failure to consider Boerhaave's syndrome in the differential diagnosis of chest and abdominal pain (see below)

Differential Diagnosis of Boerhaave's Syndrome

- Acute myocardial infarction
- Pulmonary embolism
- Acute pancreatitis
- Acute cholecystitis
- Spontanous pneumothorax

Investigations for Boerhaave's Syndrome

1. Chest X-ray is normal in 10 to 12% of the patients. Positive findings include surgical or mediastinal emphysema (which

may take 1 hour to develop), pneumothorax or hydropneumothorax, and pleural effusion (usually on the left, occasionally bilateral).

2. Radiocontrast oesophageogram using gastrographin is positive in up to 75% of the patients, while negative results are due to the perforation being blocked by food, oedema, or clot. Never use barium in suspected ruptured oesophagus.

3. Thoracocentesis of the pleural effusion. Boerhaave's syndrome is suggested by an acidic pleural fluid (pH < 6), or the presence of food in the pleural effusion.

4. CT scan of the chest.

Management of Boerhaave's Syndrome

The delay in making the diagnosis is associated with increasing mortality as follows:

- 12 hours delay in diagnosis   mortality = 36%
- 24 hours delay in diagnosis   mortality = 64%

These patients require ITU care and urgent referral for surgery. The operative approach is not contraindicated by the presence of shock. In the pre-operative period, the patient is kept nil by mouth, and supported with intravenous fluids, broad-spectrum antibiotics and appropriate oxygenation. Without surgical intervention, Boerhaave's syndrome is usually incompatible with life. Therefore, the conservative approach is reserved for those patients with small oesophageal tears and late diagnosis.

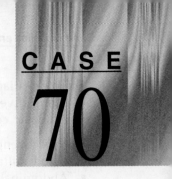

C A S E
70

CASE 70

A 65-year-old man with a past medical history of constipation presented with upper abdominal pain and fever. He had been on holiday five weeks ago to southern Italy and developed diarrhea for a few days. His General Practitioner treated him with antibiotics and the symptoms settled. He lived alone and did not smoke cigarettes or drink alcohol. On examination, his temperature was 38.4° Celsius, pulse 96 bpm regular, and blood pressure 160/95 mmHg. The descending colon was palpable and tender. The liver was tender and enlarged to 4 cm below the right costal margin. He was admitted to hospital and continued to have intermittent fever (37.5° to 39.5° Celsius). His initial investigations were:

ESR	72 mm/h
Hb	10.2 g/l
MCV	100 fl
MCH	31 pg
WBC	10.4 × 10⁹/l
Neutrophils	80%
Bilirubin	32 µmol/l
AST	180 U/l
ALT	438 U/l
ALP	270 U/l
Urine	Trace protein
CXR	Small right basal effusion and left apical fibrosis

Questions
1. What is the differential diagnosis?
2. Name six important investigations.

Answers

1. The main diagnostic possibilities are:
   - Acute diverticulitis and liver abscess
   - Amoebic colitis and liver abscess

2. The six essential investigations are:
   - Blood cultures
   - Abdominal ultrasound or CT scan
   - Stool examination for Entamoeba histolytica
   - Stool cultures
   - Viral hepatitis serology screen
   - Diagnostic pleural aspiration

Constipation, abdominal pain, fever and leucocytosis could be diverticulitis, which may be complicated by a paracolic abscess or liver abscess. The tender hepatomegaly and abnormal LFTs could be either hepatitis or liver abscess. The episode of diarrhoea while on holiday has many possible causes, such as E. coli, Shigella, Salmonella, Giardia, or Entamoeba. Amoebic liver abscess can develop insidiously without much in the way of bowel symptoms. The left apical fibrosis suggests old pulmonary tuberculosis (TB) that may have re-activated. Active TB alone would not explain all his symptoms i.e. diarrhoea and evidence of acute hepatitis or liver abscess. Gastrointestinal malignancy with superadded intra-abdominal sepsis would remain a diagnostic possibility.

This patient's fever was unexplained over a five-week period. Clinicians should have a systematic approach to patients with pyrexia of unknown origin (PUO). The criteria for defining PUO includes:
- Fever has persisted for 3 or more weeks
- Routine clinical and laboratory investigations have failed to demonstrate an underlying cause during this time

Body temperature is controlled by the hypothalamus through different types of responses including the following:
1. Autonomic
2. Somatic
3. Endocrine (catecholamines and thyroxine increase body temperature)
4. Behavioural

The hypothalamus contains thermostatic controls that encourage heat production or heat loss. Heat production is due to muscular activity, basal metabolic rate, and specific dynamic action (heat obtained by food ingestion). The heat loss is achieved by:

- Radiation and conduction   70%
- Vaporisation of sweat   27%
- Respiration   2%
- Urination and defecation   1%

Causes of Pyrexia of Unknown Origin (PUO)

1. Many bacterial infections can present as PUO, but look particularly for:
    - Bacterial endocarditis
    - Intra-abdominal abscess: sub-phrenic, pelvic, renal, perinephric, retroperitoneal
    - Chronic septicaemia: meningococcal
    - Tuberculosis (TB), such as miliary, gastrointestinal, spinal, renal, pelvic
    - Brucellosis
    - Typhoid
    - Leptospirosis
    - Viral and rickettsial infections: Q fever, infectious mononucleosis
    - Protozoal disease: malaria, amoebic liver disease, kala-azar, trypanosomiasis, histoplasmosis, toxoplasmosis
2. Maliganancy: lymphoma, leukaemia, carcinomatosis, hypernephroma, hepatoma.
3. Chronic granulomatous conditions: Crohn's disease, sarcoidosis
4. Vasculitis: SLE, polyarteritis nodosa, Still's disease, giant cell arteritis, polymyalgia rheumatica.
5. Familial Mediterranean fever
6. Drug induced fever
7. Factitious fever

This list is not comprehensive and some conditions are more common in some parts of the world.

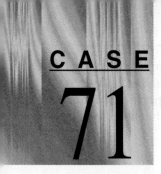

C A S E

71

CASE 71

An 83-year-old woman with a past medical history of hypertension, basal cell carcinoma of the right temple treated with local radiotherapy, and osteoarthritis of the knees presented with severe pain in the left leg, pain and stiffness in the hips, thighs, shoulders, and upper back. Her initial ESR was 34 mm/h. A diagnosis of polymyalgia rheumatica was made and she improved with steroids. Her ESR fell to 20 mm/h. Seven months later she was referred to the rheumatology clinic with severe pain in the right shoulder, left arm, and interscapular region precipitated by movement. On examination, there was tenderness in the upper thoracic spine and right shoulder. The left breast showed an ulcerative tumour, but there were no enlarged lymph nodes. She was commenced on tamoxifen. Six days later she developed weakness of both legs, became unable to walk, and had difficulty in passing urine. Cranial nerves were intact and arms were normal in power, sensation, and reflexes. Both legs were weak with a power 3/5 and reflexes were exaggerated. There was also reduced pinprick sensation up to the thighs, reduced vibration in the right leg, and reduced proprioception at the great toe. Both plantar reflexes were extensor.

Hb	13.5 g/dl	WBC	$12.0 \times 10^9/l$
Platelet	$329 \times 10^9/l$	MCV	92.5 fl
MCHC	32.9 g/dl	Na	138 mmol/l
K	3.4 mmol/l	Urea	7.7 mmol/l
Creatinine	100 µmol/l	Glucose	13.0 mmol/l
Bilirubin	10 µmol/l	Albumin	42 g/l
ALT	18 U/l	ALP	118 U/l
Corrected calcium	2.44 mmol/l	PO_4	0.91 mmol/l

Questions
1. What is the likely diagnosis?
2. Give two imaging investigations.

Answers

1. Spastic paraparesis due to malignant cord compression.
2. MRI scan of the spine and isotope bone scan.

The MRI showed a combination of vertebral collapse and cord compression at the levels T2, T3, T5 and T7. The isotope bone scan showed multiple metastatic deposits.

Anatomy of the Spinal Cord

- The spinal cord extends from the foramina magnum to the level of L1 spine
- The cord is covered by both arachnoid and dura maters
- The stability of the cord within the canal is maintained by the two denticulate ligaments which join the cord to the dura mater on each lateral side
- The anterior side of the spinal canal is covered by the ligamentum flavum
- The line between the two iliac crests pass through the space between the L3 and L4 vertebrae
- The spinous processes do not exactly match with the cord segments

Causes of Flaccid Weakness in the Legs

- Guillain-Barré syndrome
- Acute intermittent porphyria
- Lead poisoning
- Thallium poisoning
- Myopathies and muscular dystrophies
- Cauda equina lesion

Causes of Spastic Weakness in the Legs

- Cord compression
- Bilateral cerebrovascular disease
- Multiple sclerosis
- Transverse myelitis
- Subacute combined degeneration of the cord
- Motor neurone disease (amyotrophic lateral sclerosis)
- Syringomyelia
- Spinal vascular disease i.e. spinal cord infarction
- Falx meningioma

Causes of Spinal Cord Compression
- Neoplastic
- Cervical myelopathy
- Disc prolapse and spondylosis
- Trauma
- Epidural abscess
- Pott's disease (tuberculous spondylitis)
- Epidural haemorrhage

Spastic Paraparesis and Diagnostic Clinical Signs

The following clinical signs are diagnostically useful in establishing the aetiology of spastic paraparesis.

Presence of cerebellar signs suggest:
- Multiple sclerosis
- Malignancy

Wasted hand muscles and spastic paraparesis suggest:
- Cervical spondylosis
- Cervical cord tumour (at the C8/T1 level)
- Syringomyelia
- Motor neurone disease

Absent knee jerks and extensor plantars suggest:
- Subacute combined degeneration of the cord with polyneuropathy due to vitamin B_{12} deficiency
- Motor neurone disease (amyotrophic lateral sclerosis). Look for muscle wasting and fasciculations
- Diabetic polyneuropathy and cervical spondylosis
- Neurosyphilis: the combination of tabes dorsalis and general paralysis of the insane (GPI) is called taboparesis
- Friedreich's ataxia

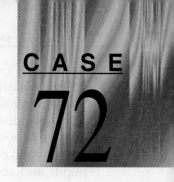

C A S E

72

CASE 72

A 75-year-old lady was admitted to hospital with confusion. The family noticed that she has lost the sight in both eyes and bumped into walls and objects in all directions. She was normally self-caring. The optometrist had checked her vision recently and she needed reading spectacles. Her only past medical problem had been hypertension, which was treated with a thiazide diuretic. On examination, she had multiple bruises over the face and right arm. The pupils were equal at 4 mm and reacted normally to light. Fundoscopy was normal. She was not aware that she had lost her vision and could not even perceive light. There was no dysarthria, nystagmus, or ophthalmoplegia. There was no focal weakness, the reflexes were symmetrical, and the plantars were flexor. The blood pressure was elevated (182/98 mmHg) and the heart was in sinus rhythm. There were no signs of valvular heart disease or cardiac failure. The carotid and femoral arterial pulses were palpable and without audible bruits.

Questions
1. What investigation would you request to establish the diagnosis?
2. What is the differential diagnosis?

Answers

1. CT brain scan.
2. The differential diagnosis includes: a) bilateral cortical blindness due to cerebral oedema or stroke; b) toxic damage to optic nerves due to alcohol poisoning; c) cranial arteritis; and d) functional blindness. However, the normal pupils and absence of primary retinal pathology should alert the clinician to the diagnosis of cortical blindness.

Cortical Blindness

In this patient CT scan of the brain showed ischaemic infarction in both occipital lobes, i.e. bilateral occipital stroke. Cortical blindness is the loss of vision due to damage to both occipital lobes, or both optic radiations beyond the lateral geniculate body. The classic triad of cortical blindness includes:

• Bilateral blindness
• Normal fundi
• Intact pupillary light reflexes.

Some patients deny blindness and this is known as Anton's syndrome. The commonest cause of cortical blindness is a stroke. The blindness may be incomplete or complete and this depends on the extent of cortical damage.

The retinal fibres run through the optic nerve, optic chiasma and optic tract and synapse at the lateral geniculate body. The optic fibres from the lateral geniculate body pass in the optic radiation through the temporal and the parietal lobes to reach the visual cortex in the occipital lobe. However, the afferent fibres that participate in the pupillary light reflex bypass the lateral geniculate body and end in the pretectal area of the midbrain. From here the impulses are relayed to the Edinger-Westphal nucleus. Efferent fibres from the Edinger-Westphal nucleus pass through the third (oculo-motor) nerve to reach the ciliary ganglion and finally reach the pupil. Hence pupillary reflexes are spared in cortical lesions and the fundi look normal. The posterior cerebral artery (PCA) supplies the visual cortex and PCA occlusions are commonly caused by an embolus.

CASE 73

A 68-year-old lady presented with diplopia and weakness of the right arm and leg. She had been a diabetic and hypertensive for the past 20 years. On examination, she had a right hemiparesis. There was drooping of the left eyelid, the left eye was deviated laterally, and the left pupil was dilated. Diplopia occurred on looking to the right side.

Questions
1. What is the diagnosis?
2. What investigation would you request to establish the diagnosis?

Answers
1. Weber's syndrome
2. CT brain to exclude haemorrhage followed by MRI scan of the brain to demonstrate the ischaemic lesion in the midbrain.

Weber's Syndrome

The German physician Hermann Weber described Weber's syndrome in 1863. The lesion is located in the midbrain (crus cerebri) and the clinical findings include ipsilateral third nerve palsy and contralateral limb weakness.

The third nerve nuclei are located in the midbrain and extend up to 10 mm in length from the rostral to caudal extent. It consists of two groups of nuclei:
1. Edinger-Westphal nucleus in the upper midbrain and supplies fibres to the pupils.
2. Motor nucleus in the lower midbrain and supplies the extraocular muscles, except the lateral rectus and the superior oblique.

Fibres from the nuclei run forward and laterally through the red nuclei, converge at the interpeduncular fossa and emerge from the midbrain. The nuclei and fascicles in the mid-brain are spread across a wide area and hence midbrain lesions (intra-axial) can lead to partial third nerve lesions. A lesion of the lower midbrain affects the extra-ocular muscles, but spares the pupils, whereas lesions involving both upper and lower parts of the midbrain cause pupillary dilatation. Emerging from the midbrain, the third nerve lies between the posterior cerebral artery and superior cerebellar artery and runs forward parallel to the posterior communicating artery. It then enters the orbit through the superior orbital fissure and divides into upper and lower branches. The upper branch supplies the superior rectus muscle and the levator palpebrae superioris. The lower branch supplies three ocular muscles: the medial rectus, the inferior rectus, and the inferior oblique. The nerve to the inferior oblique muscle carries the preganglionic parasympathetic fibres to the ciliary ganglion. The postganglionic parasympathetic fibres arise from here to supply the ciliary muscle and the muscles of the iris (pupilloconstrictor fibres).

The pupilloconstrictor fibres and those innervating the levator palpebrae lie in a superficial and dorsal position on the nerve relaying in the ciliary ganglion, which is in the posterior orbit. Because of this anatomical characteristic, a fixed dilated pupil is often the first sign of third nerve compression and ptosis the second before external ophthalmoplegia develops. Pupil sparing third nerve palsy can also occur with lesions affecting the nerve trunk (extra-axial lesions) as in ischaemic damage to the third nerve and diabetes mellitus.

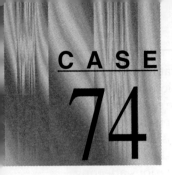

CASE

74

CASE 74

A 75-year-old man was admitted with a history of shortness of breath and non-productive cough. On systemic enquiry he had been "generally unwell" over the last 4 months with lethargy, poor appetite, and 4 kg weight loss. There was no other past medical history. He was not on any regular medications, did not smoke cigarettes, or drink alcohol. He retired after working for 35 years as a chemical engineer, lived with his wife, and has three children. Clinically he was thinly built. There was no pallor or jaundice. Both legs were oedematous. His blood pressure was 196/98 mmHg and pulse 84 bpm regular. The initial blood tests were as follows:

Hb	10 g/dl
WBC	$7.2 \times 10^9/l$
Platelets	$352 \times 10^9/l$
MCV	86.1 fl
MCH	30.5 pg
MCHC	35.4 g/dl
Na	147 mmol/l
K	2.5 mmol/l
Urea	6.5 mmol/l
Creatinine	63 µmol/l
Glucose	6.0 mmol/l
CRP	70 mg/l
Bilirubin	38 µmol/l
ALT	40 U/l
ALP	95 U/l

Questions
1. What is the most likely diagnosis?
2. Name six investigations.

Answers

1. ACTH secreting tumour
2. The relevant investigations are:
   a. CXR
   b. Plasma cortisol
   c. 24 hour urinary cortisol
   d. Dexamethasone suppression test
   e. Plasma ACTH level
   f. Ultrasound or CT scan of the abdomen

The positive findings were hypertension and hypokalaemia on the background of poor appetite and weight loss. Unfortunately, these findings were not tied together diagnostically on admission. These features should always alert the clinician to the diagnosis of excessive production of corticosteroid or mineralocorticoid hormones. This gentleman's urinary free cortisol was elevated at 1,311 nmol/day (ref 50-180) and plasma ACTH level was also elevated 382 ng/l (ref 10-80). In Cushing's syndrome due to an ectopic source of ACTH severe cachexia and marked hypokalaemia are typical features. Ultrasound of the abdomen in this patient showed multiple metastatic nodules and the liver biopsy was consistent with a small cell carcinoma.

Cushing's Syndrome

Cushing's syndrome could be ACTH-dependent or non-ACTH-dependent.

ACTH Dependent

- Pituitary adenoma (Cushing's disease)
- Ectopic ACTH-producing tumours of lung, pancreatic tumours, carcinoid tumours, medullary thyroid carcinoma, and phaeochromocytoma
- ACTH use

Non-ACTH Dependent

- Adrenal adenomas and carcinomas
- Corticosteroid use

Diagnostic Workup in Suspected Cushing's Syndrome

In a case of suspected Cushing's syndrome the aims are:

-243-

1. Establish the presence of hypercortisolaemia

In Cushing's syndrome there is excessive cortisol production with loss of the normal circadian rhythm. For in-patients midnight plasma cortisol above 50 nmol/l and an elevated urinary free cortisol are useful markers of excessive cortisol secretion (normal range = 50-180 nmol/day). The overnight dexamethasone is useful in out-patients: 1 mg of dexamethasone is given at midnight and the plasma cortisol measured at 09.00 hours should be < 50 nmol/l in normal subjects.

2. Establish its cause and proceed with treatment

The following investigations may elucidate the cause of Cushing's syndrome:

- 09.00h ACTH levels (reference range 10-80 ng/l)
  In pituitary Cushing's ACTH levels could be normal, slightly elevated or high: typical ACTH range < 50 to 250 ng/l.
  In Cushing's syndrome from ectopic ACTH levels are generally very high: >200 ng/l, but the typical range is < 80 to >12,000 ng/l and, therefore, overlaps greatly with pituitary Cushing's syndrome.
  In adrenal causes of Cushing's syndrome ACTH levels are usually low (< 10 ng/l) or undetectable.
- High dose dexamethasone test: 2 mg of dexamethasone is given 6 hourly for 48 hours. Urine and plasma cortisols should fall by 50%. This response is expected in 80% of patients with Cushing's disease (i.e. pituitary adenoma producing excess ACTH) and 20% of patients with ectopic ACTH.
- Corticotropin releasing hormone (CRH) test
  In pituitary-dependent Cushing's syndrome, in response to 100mg of CRH administered IV, levels of ACTH levels rise by 50%.
- Inferior petrosal sinus sampling of plasma ACTH after intravenous CRH
  This test will differentiate between pituitary dependent disease and ectopic ACTH, but is only available in specialist centres. In pituitary disease the ACTH level from the inferior petrosal sinus will be many times higher than that in the peripheral vein. The ratio of ACTH in the

inferior petrosal sinus divided by that in the peripheral vein of > 3 suggests pituitary adenoma.

- Imaging: pituitary CT or MRI, adrenal CT or MRI. Beware that some healthy people will have a pituitary incidentaloma. This situation is described elsewhere in this book.

Differential Diagnosis of Hypertension with Hypokalaemia

- Essential hypertension and diuretic therapy (the most common cause)
- Cushing's syndrome
- Conn's syndrome
- Liquorice consumption in large amounts
- Liddle's syndrome (low aldosterone). There is an increased sodium-potassium exchange and the condition responds to triamterene.

Bartter's Syndrome

This condition was first described by Bartter in 1962 among two patients of African origin. They had hypokalaemic alkalosis, pitressin-resistant diabetes insipidus and secondary hyperaldosteronism *without hypertension*.

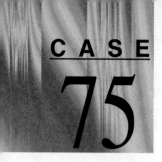

C A S E

75

CASE 75

A 76-year-old lady presented to the A&E department with sudden severe occipital headache of three hours duration. She was not on any medications and apart from cholecystectomy, there was no other past medical history. She drank alcohol occasionally and smoked 20 cigarettes a day. On examination, she was alert and her BP was 174/88 mmHg and pulse 76 bpm regular. The heart, chest, and abdomen were unremarkable. There was complete left sided ptosis, which had appeared in the last few hours. On lifting the left upper eye, the left pupil was dilated and there was a divergent squint. The right eye was normal. She was uncomfortable with the movement of the neck. While the medical officer was writing up the clinical history, the nurse alerted him that his patient was deteriorating. She had become drowsy and could not move her right arm and leg.

Question
1. What is the diagnosis?
2. List the most important two measures in her management.

Answers

1. Subarachnoid haemorrhage (SAH) due to rupture of aneurysm of the posterior communicating artery
2. Urgent CT scan of the head and referral to the neurosurgical department

Subarachnoid Haemorrhage

The incidence of SAH is about 10-15 per 100,000 in the Western World. The most common cause of SAH is ruptured arterial aneurysms, which is responsible for 75% of cases. The second most common cause is ruptured arteriovenous (AV) malformation, which accounts for about 15% of the patients with SAH. Other causes include bleeding diathesis, anticoagulant therapy, bleeding from tumours and vasculitis. In about 15% of the patients, the cause of the SAH remains unidentified.

The intracranial vessels lie in the subarachnoid space and give off perforating branches to the brain tissue. SAH is usually due to bleeding from these vessels, although in some patients SAH may result from ruptured intracerebral aneurysms that usually present as primary intracerebral haemorrhage (PICH). The main symptom of SAH is headache, which is of abrupt onset, and usually described as a "blow to the head". This is sometimes preceded by a few mild attacks of headache or "warning leaks". Epileptic seizures or loss of consciousness may follow the headache. The signs of meningism develop 3-12 hours after the onset of the SAH and the main signs are neck stiffness and Kernig's sign. Many patients also develop focal neurological signs such as hermiplegia or dysphasia due to intracerebral collection of blood or vasospasm. Patients may also show reactive hypertension with or without pyrexia. Examination of the fundus may reveal papilloedema, subhyaloid haemorhage, or vitreous haemorrahge.

Diagnosis of SAH

1. CT scan of the head
2. Lumbar puncture (LP).
   Note: the contraindications to LP.

- CT scan usually confirms the diagnosis of SAH in 95% of the cases if it is done within 48 hours. When the scan is positive, the blood may be seen widespread in the basal cisterns and interhemispheric fissure with or without intraventricular extension. However, the bleeding could be more localized to the site of the ruptured aneurysm, such as the sylvian fissure from middle cerebral artery or interhemispheric fissure due to ruptured anterior communicating artery. Free blood may also be seen over the cortical sulci.
- In addition the CT scan may reveal associated abnormalities such as:
  1. Hydrocephalus
  2. Intracerebral haemorrhage
  3. Tumours
  4. AV malformations
- If the CT scan is negative, LP is indicated provided that more than 6 hours has elapsed from the onset of the SAH, and that the patient is alert (i.e. no disturbance of consciousness) and has no focal neurological signs.
- If the CSF is clear, it is subjected to spectrophotometry, but xanthochromia takes at least six hours to develop.

Strategies for the Management of SAH

- If the CT scan is negative and the CSF is clear, then no further action is required
- However, if the CT scan is positive and the patient is alert without focal signs, referral to the neurosurgical unit should be under 12 hours. Urgent referral is indicated in those with focal neurological signs or disturbed consciousness.

Neurological Complications of SAH

- Rebleeding
- Cerebral ischaemia and infarction
- Hydrocephalus
- Expanding haematoma
- Epilepsy

Non-neurological Complications of SAH

- Acute myocardial infarction
- Cardiac arrhythmias
- Acute pulmonary oedema
- Reactive hypertension
- Gastric ulcer (stress ulcer) with or without bleeding
- Reduced plasma volume
- Hyponatraemia
- Pyrexia

Rebleeding after the SAH

In untreated patients with SAH, rebleeding occurs in about 30% of the patients in the first 28 days. Among those who survive, rebleeding occurs in another 20% in the subsequent 5 months. The risk of rebleeding remains significant even among the survivors after the first six months. When rebleeding occurs, it appears as SAH but usually the headache is more severe.

Cerebral Ischaemia and Infarction

Cerebral ischaemia leading to cerebral infarction is common after SAH and it may occur immediately, or typically it is delayed until the period between the 4th and the 12th day after the onset of the SAH. Vasospastic agents released from the vessel walls or blood clots are thought to be responsible for the vasospasm. It is estimated that cerebral ischaemia occurs in 25% of the patients and among these about 25% will die. About 10% of the survivors who are complicated by cerebral ischaemia leading to cerebral infarction will remain severely dependent.

Hypovolumia after SAH

After the SAH, there is increased urinary sodium excretion leading to hypovolumia. This is different from the syndrome of inappropriate antidiuretic secretion. The reduced plasma volume may directly affect the cerebral perfusion, but the hyperviscosity may lead to cerebral thrombosis and ischaemia.

Cerebral perfusion pressure = mean systolic pressure – intracranial pressure

Hydrocephalus after SAH

They are of two types:
1. Obstructive hydrocephalus due to blood clots in the ventricular system
2. Non-obstructive (communicating type), which may be due to blood clots within the basal cisterns or obstruction of the arachnoid villi.

Hydrocephalus should be suspected in any patient with SAH who develops one or more of the following:
- Headache
- Deterioration of consciousness
- Impairment of cognitive function
- Incontinence
- Gait ataxia

Medical Management of SAH

1. Bed rest
2. Pain relief: paracetamol, codeine or dihydrocodeine. Avoid strong opiates
3. Calcium channel blockers (nimodipine or nicardipine) to prevent cerebral vasospasm
4. Avoidance of antihypertensive medication. In normal subjects, a fall in blood pressure leads to cerebral vasodilatation, which maintains the cerebral perfusion, and this is called cerebral autoregulation. However, the latter is often impaired in patients with SAH and as a result, any fall in blood pressure leads to reduced cerebral perfusion with subsequent cerebral ischaemia and infarction.
5. High fluid intake. It is recommended that patients with SAH should at least take 3 litres of fluid per day to prevent hypovolumia. If the serum sodium falls < 130 mmol/l, fluids should not be restricted, but fludrocortisone or hypertonic saline should be given instead. These are better guided through plasma and urinary assessments of sodium and osmolality along with the central venous pressure measurements.

Plasma Volume Expansion

High-risk patients and those who show the first sign of cerebral ischaemia should be given plasma expanders, but if they deteriorate blood pressure should be raised by inotropes.

Outcome and Prognosis of SAH

Mortality from SAH and dependency among the survivors are quite high. Predictors for increased mortality are depressed level of consciousness, advanced age, thickness of the subarachnoid hemorrhage clot on computerized tomography, elevated blood pressure, pre-existing medical illnesses, and basilar aneurysms. The mortality at six months is shown in the Table.

Table: Management Mortality after SAH at Six Months*

State of consciousness on admission	Number of patients	Mortality (%)	Good recovery (%)
Alert	1722	13%	74%
Drowsy	1136	28%	54%
Stuporose	348	44%	30%
Comatose	315	72%	11%

* Kassell NF, Torner JC, Haley Jr EC, Jane JA, Adams HP, Kongable GL. Journal of Neurosurgery 1990; 73: 18-36. Stuporose = severely depressed arousal with some response to vigorous stimuli. Comatose = total or near total unresponsiveness.

SAH and Third Nerve Palsy

The differential diagnoses are:

1. Rupture of aneurysm of the posterior communicating artery. Emerging from the midbrain, the third nerve lies between the posterior cerebral artery and superior cerebellar artery and runs forward parallel to the posterior communicating artery.
2. SAH and transtentorial herniation
3. Ruptured aneurysm of basilar artery (very rare and fatal).

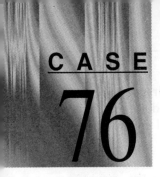

CASE 76

A 24-year-old man was referred to the cardiology clinic with a six months history of recurrent palpitations. They usually lasted only a few seconds or minutes and subsided spontaneously. There were no definite precipitating factors and the palpitations seemed to come on even at rest. There was no significant past medical history. He worked as a trainee in an automobile shop, did not smoke, and drank two to three pints of beer at weekends. He has an elder sister who was well. An ECG was done and is shown below.

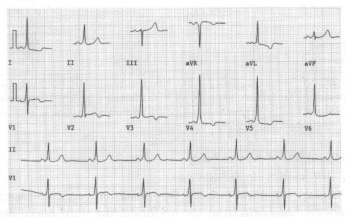

Question
What is the diagnosis?

Answer

Type A Wolff-Parkinson-White (WPW) syndrome

Wolff-Parkinson-White (WPW) Syndrome

WPW syndrome is a pre-excitation syndrome wherein the presence of an accessory pathway between the atria and ventricles activates the ventricular myocardium prematurely. This accessory pathway, which is called the bundle of Kent, conducts the atrial impulses to the ventricle without any AV nodal delay resulting in a short PR interval. The 'delta' wave is due to slower conduction in the area of ordinary myocardium separating the bundle of Kent and the His Purkinje system. Once the electrical impulse has reached the His Purkinje system, rapid conduction ensues and the remainder of the R wave is normal in configuration.

The accessory pathways have been described at many different sites along the atrioventricular (AV) groove, but the most commonly known types of WPW syndrome are types A and B. In type A the accessory pathway is situated between the posterior left atrial wall and the left ventricle. The ECG shows a positive 'delta' wave in lead V1 in type A WPW. In type B the accessory pathway is situated between the lateral right atrial wall and the right ventricle. The ECG shows a biphasic or negative 'delta' wave in lead V1 in type B WPW.

The ECG findings of WPW syndrome cause difficulties with other ECG diagnoses as follows:

ECG Differential Diagnosis of Type A WPW syndrome

- Right bundle branch block (RBBB)
- Right ventricular hypertrophy (RVH)
- True posterior myocardial infarction

ECG Differential Diagnosis of Type B WPW syndrome

- Left Bundle Branch Block
- Q wave pattern (negative delta wave) in lead aVF with a pseudo-infarction pattern in the inferior leads.

WPW syndrome usually occurs as an isolated cardiac anomaly, but may co-exist with other conditions such as:
- Ebstein's anomaly

- Hypertrophic obstructive cardiomyopathy
- Mitral valve prolapse

Complications of WPW syndrome

- Atrial fibrillation (AF)

  AF in WPW is usually conducted through the bundle of Kent and, therefore, the delta wave is seen in the QRS complexes. The ventricular rate in AF due to WPW syndrome is usually fast, which may cause cardiovascular collapse and degenerate to ventricular fibrillation. In this condition, one must not use digoxin or AV nodal suppressing agents as they may accelerate the conduction through the accessory pathway and the patient will become worse. The safest way to terminate AF due to WPW syndrome is electrical cardioversion, but if drugs are to be used the choices are for IV disopyramide or flecainide. Intravenous amiodarone is dangerous unless given over 1-4 hours. AF with a very fast ventricular rate should always alert the clinician to the possibility of underlying WPW syndrome.

- AV re-entrant tachycardia and AV nodal re-entrant tachycardia

  Here, the AV junction and the bundle of Kent differ in the time that they take to recover. Usually the AV junction recovers first. A premature atrial ectopic beat during sinus rhythm while the AV junction has recovered and the bundle of Kent is refractory will be transmitted to the ventricles. When the bundle of Kent has recovered, it is able to transmit the atrial premature beat retrogradely to the atria. If the cycle is repeated, a circuit tachycardia is produced. The ECG during AV re-entrant tachycardia will show regular and narrow ventricular complexes unless phasic aberrant conduction occurs. The QRS complexes do not show the delta waves. The P waves (if seen) are usually midway between the QRS complexes (see diagram). In some individuals there is an additional pathway *within the AV node,* which allows retrograde conduction and a circuit for tachycardia. This is called *AV nodal re-entrant tachycardia,* and the P waves are inverted and seen immediately after the QRS complexes (see diagram).

Vagal manoeuvres may terminate AV re-entrant tachycardia. If they are ineffective, the options are electrical cardioversion if the patient is haemodynamically unstable, or drugs such as IV disopyramide, flecainide, or ajmaline. For the long-term prophylaxis of WPW tachycardias, beta blockers, flecainide, disopyramide, or amiodarone could be used. Digoxin and verapamil are contraindicated.

Concealed Bundle of Kent

In these patients the accessory pathway is only capable of conduction from the ventricles to the atria and hence the surface ECG during the sinus rhythm does not show the delta waves.

Wolff-Parkinson-White AV Re-entrant Tachycardia

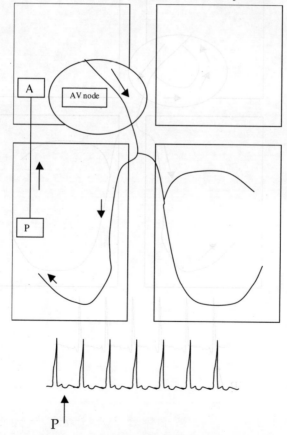

- Anterograde conduction down the AV node *and* retrograde conduction up the Accessory Pathway (AP)
- There are narrow QRS complexes
- There is no delta wave
- Inverted P wave is seen after the QRS, usually midway between QRS complexes.

Note:
- Anterograde conduction down the Accessory Pathway *and* retrograde conduction up the AV node is rare
- In this situation the delta wave is present

Wolff-Parkinson-White AV Nodal Re-entrant Tachycardia

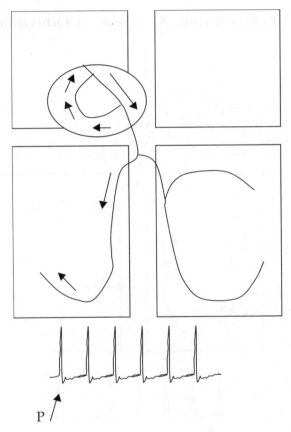

- There is an additional pathway *within* the AV node.
- Anterograde conduction down the normal AV nodal pathway
  and retrograde conduction via the abnormal additional pathway.
- Inverted P waves are often difficult to detect and occur immediately after the QRS complexes.

Lown-Ganong-Levine syndrome

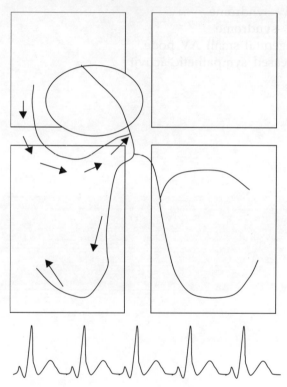

- The accessory pathway is called the bundle of James and connects directly with the Bundle of His
- There is no delta wave
- The PR interval is shortened (less than 0.08 seconds)

Lown-Ganong-Levine (LGL) Syndrome

This is a pre-excitation syndrome due to the presence of an additional accessory pathway between the atrial myocardium and the bundle of His. Therefore, an atrial impulse will reach the ventricles without the normal delay and lead to a short PR interval. The ECG will not show a delta wave as the atrial impulse is conducted to the ventricle through the bundle of His and Purkinje system. These patients are prone to AV re-entrant tachycardia and are treated in the same way as those arising from WPW syndrome.

Causes of a Short PR Interval

1. WPW syndrome
2. LGL syndrome
3. Congenital small AV node
4. Increased sympathetic activity

CASE

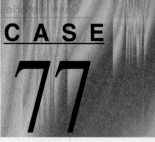

CASE 77

A 43-year-old lady was attending the endocrine clinic for the follow-up of Hashimoto's thyroiditis. Routine liver function tests (LFTs) showed:

Bilirubin	9 μmol/l
AST	184 U/l
ALT	248 U/l
ALP	88 U/l
γ-GT	62 U/l
Total protein	89 g/l
Albumin	43 g/l

Questions
1. What is the most likely diagnosis?
2. List five important investigations

Answers
1. Chronic active hepatitis (lupoid type)
2. Five important investigation should include:
   Viral hepatitis screen (B, C, D)
   Autoantibodies
   Abdominal ultrasound
   Coagulation screen
   Liver biopsy

This patient has normal bilirubin, alkaline phosphatase and albumin levels. However, there was evidence of hepatocellular damage as indicated by raised AST, ALT and γ-GT. The hepatocellular damage is mild and associated with increased globulins suggesting a chronic inflammatory process. After two weeks the following results became available:

Antinuclear factor	weakly positive
Smooth muscle antibody	strongly positive
Antimitochondrial antibody	negative
Viral screen for Hepatitis B, C and D	negative
Coagulation screen	normal
Abdominal ultrasound	mildly enlarged liver without focal lesion
Liver biopsy	piece meal necrosis compatible with chronic active hepatitis

She was started on steroids and azathioprine. After 10 months the LFTs were as follows:

Bilirubin	10 μmol/l
AST	26 U/l
ALT	35 U/l
ALP	58 U/l
γ-GT	52 U/l
Total protein	73 g/l
Albumin	42 g/l

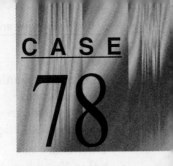
CASE 78

A 36-year-old gentleman was referred to the medical out patients department because of aches and pains in the limbs. He had been epileptic for over 20 years and drank alcohol excessively. The control of epilepsy had been poor in the past six months with grand mal seizures occurring almost weekly. He was taking phenytoin 250 mg od. On examination, there was no focal neurological deficit. The following results became available:

Albumin	30 g/l
Calcium	1.8 mmol/l
Phosphate	0.6 mmol/l
Bilirubin	18 µmol/l
AST	24 U/l
ALT	38 U/l
ALP	720 U/l

Questions
1. What are the major biochemical abnormalities?
2. Suggest two clinical diagnoses

Answers

1. Hypocalcaemia, hypophosphataemia and raised alkaline phosphatase.
2. Osteomalacia secondary to poor diet or chronic anti-convulsive therapy.

The history of excessive alcohol intake makes a primary alcohol induced hepatic problem a possibility. However, the AST and ALT were normal and he was not jaundiced. The raised ALP may occur in asymptomatic primary biliary cirrhosis, hepatic infiltration with malignancy, or granulomatous disease. In this patient the isoenzymes of the ALP showed that it was from bony origin. Indeed an ultrasound examination of the liver was normal. A detailed history showed inadequate dietary intake, which along with the chronic use of phenytoin was the presumed cause of osteomalacia. The latter diagnosis was confirmed by bone biopsy.

Side Effects from Chronic Use of Phenytoin

- Gingival hypertrophy, acne, hirsutism, and coarse facial features
- Folate deficiency
- Polyneuroapthy
- Lymphadenopathy (pseudolymphoma)
- Rickets and osteomalacia

Side Effects of Over Dosage of Phenytoin

- Nausea and vomiting
- Confusion
- Ataxia (both low and high levels can cause ataxia and poor control of epilepsy)
- Tremor and nystagmus
- Headache
- Slurred speech
- Blurred vision

Other Side Effects of Phenytoin

- Bone marrow dyscrasia
- Stevens-Johnson syndrome; toxic epidermal necrolysis

- Fever and hepatitis
- Connective tissue disorders including SLE and polyarteritis nodosa.

For detailed discussion of the adverse effects of phenytoin, please consult the manufacturer's data sheet or a standard pharmacology textbook.

CASE 79

A 58-year-old man presented to the casualty department with acute onset central chest pain radiating to the left arm. He was not taking any medications. He smoked about 40 cigarettes per day. There were no previous problems with diabetes and cardiac or respiratory disease. He worked as a builder and lived with his wife and 3 children. His elder brother aged 68 was also a heavy smoker and suffered from ischaemic heart disease over the last 2 years. On examination, he was in sinus rhythm and his blood pressure was 82/54 mmHg. The chest was clear. The medical registrar reviewed him and found that the jugular venous pressure was markedly raised. The ECG for this patient is shown below:

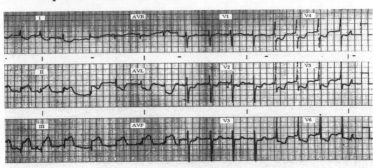

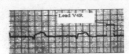

Question
What is the ECG diagnosis?

Answer

Acute inferior myocardial infarction complicated by right ventricular infarction (RVI).

ECG Criteria in the Diagnosis of RVI

Five different ECG criteria have been suggested for the presumptive diagnosis of RVI and these include:

1. ST elevation $\geq$ 1.0 mm in leads V1-V5 without pathological Q waves in patients with acute inferior myocardial infarction (MI).
2. ST elevation $\geq$ 0.5 mm in leads V3R
3. ST elevation $\geq$ 0.5 mm in leads V4R
4. QS deflection in lead V3R
5. QS deflection in lead V4R

In the 1980's the reliability of these commonly used ECG criteria for RVI was analysed in a group 19 consecutive patients (14 men and 5 women; mean age 55 years, range 33-74) with acute inferior MI (Huwez et al). Patients with conduction defects, pericardial disease, ventricular septal defect or chronic lung disease were excluded from the study. The diagnosis of acute MI was made retrospectively in accordance with the WHO criteria. ECG's were recorded daily. *The lead V3R was recorded between V1 and V4R while lead V4R was recorded in the right midclavicular line in the 5th intercostal space.* The diagnosis of left and right ventricular infarctions were confirmed by radioisotope scans using thallium 201 and technetium 99 on days 1 and 3 from the onset of acute MI. ST segment elevations in leads V1-V3 and V3R/V4R were compared between the patients with acute inferior MI who did not have RVI and those who have had RVI.

Radionuclide studies revealed that there were 11 patients with isolated acute inferior MI and 8 patients with acute inferior MI with RVI. The ECG findings can be summarised as follows:

1. ST elevation of $\geq$ 1 mm was observed in leads V1-V3 in 2 patients with Q wave acute inferior MI and in 2 patients who had non-Q wave acute inferior MI but without RVI. However, only one patient with acute inferior MI and RVI had ST elevation $\geq$ 1 mm in leads V1-V3.
2. Patients with acute inferior MI without RVI showed ST elevation $\geq$ 0.5 mm in leads V3R and V4R in 9/11 (81%) and 2/11 (18%) respectively. Furthermore, QS waves in

leads V3R and V4R were observed in 2/11 (18%) and 4/11 (36%) respectively.

3. Patients with acute inferior MI who had RVI showed ST segment elevation ≥ 0.5 mm in leads with V3R and V4R in 6/8 (75%) and 6/8 (75%) respectively. No patient in this group showed QS waves in leads V3R while only one patient had QS waves in lead V4R.

The specificity and sensitivity of the individual ECG criteria were assessed as follows:

$$\text{Sensitivity} = \frac{\text{True positives}}{\text{True positive} + \text{False negative}} \times 100$$

$$\text{Specificity} = \frac{\text{True negatives}}{\text{True negative} + \text{False positive}} \times 100$$

Sensitivity and specificity of ST elevations for the ECG diagnosis of right ventricular infarction.

Criteria	Sensitivity	Specificity
ST elevation ≥ 1 mm in leads V1 - V3*	36%	63%
ST elevation ≥ 0.5 mm in lead V3R	75%	18%
ST elevation ≥ 0.5 mm in lead V4R	75%	81%

*ST elevation in the same leads without Q waves.

What ECG Criteria Should be Used for the Diagnosis of RVI?
In this study ST elevation ≥ 1 mm in leads V1-V3 was observed in only one patient (12%) with acute inferior MI and RVI and in about one third of those patients with acute inferior MI who did not have RVI. Therefore, the criterion of ST elevation of ≥ 1 mm in V1-V3 is of limited value in diagnosing RVI in patients with acute inferior MI. Furthermore, no patient in the RVI group has QS waves in lead V3R, but only one patient had QS deflection in lead V4R. However, the study revealed the importance of the ST elevations in V3R and V4R. Moreover, ST elevation ≥ 0.5 mm in lead V4R was significantly more frequent in patients with acute inferior MI with RVI than in those without RVI. However, there was no significant difference between these two groups with regard to ST segment elevation in lead with V3R. The criterion of

ST segment elevation ≥ 0.5 mm in lead V4R was (81%) specific for the diagnosis of RVI with a sensitivity of 75%. (see Table). The specificity of ST elevation ≥ 0.5 mm in lead with V3R was unacceptably low for the diagnosis of RVI. These results are in agreement with the findings of Klein et al (1983). They studied 58 patients who had RVI with respect to the ECG changes in lead V4R and did not report QS waves in lead V4R in a single patient. The criterion of ST elevation in lead V4R ≥ 0.5 mm was 76.9 % specific for the diagnosis of RVI with sensitivity of 82.7 %. In an editorial by Wellens (1999) the following ECG criteria in lead V4R are suggested:

1. Proximal occlusion of the right coronary artery causes ST segment elevation of at least 1 mm with positive T waves while distal occlusions produce positive T waves in lead V4R without ST segment elevation.

2. Occlusion of the circumflex artery is characterised by a negative T wave with ST depression of at least 1 mm in V4R.

Conclusions on the ECG Diagnosis of RVI

- If RVI is suspected in acute inferior MI, recordings of lead V3R and V4R should be made and examined carefully for ST elevation.

- ST elevation in lead V4R is particularly useful: ST elevation in V4R ≥ 0.5 mm has a high specificity (81%) and sensitivity (75%) for RVI.

- In patients with acute inferior MI and hypotension, we recommend an active search for the ECG features of RVI. If RVI is confirmed, effective therapy is guided by echocardiographic and haemodynamic evaluations.

References
- Huwez FU, McGhee I, Tweddel AN, Martin W, Macfarlane P. Evaluation of ST segment elevation in V1-V3 and V3R/V4R in acute inferior myocardial infarction. In: Advances in Electrocardiology, Z Antaloczy, I Preda, E Kekes (Eds.), Budapest, Hungary, Elsiever Science Publishers, 1990, 389-90.
- Klein HO, Tordjman T, Ninio R, et al. The early recognition of right ventricular infarction: diagnostic accuracy of the electrocardiographic V4R lead. Circulation 1983; 67(3): 558-65.
- Wellens, HJJ. The value of the right precordial leads of the electrocardiogram. NEJM 1999; 340(5): 381-83.

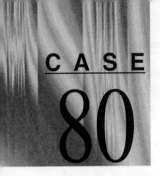

CASE 80

An 82-year-old man has deafness and headache. These are his blood test results:

Hb	12.4 g/dl
WBC	4.2 x 10⁹/l
Platelets	226 x 10⁹/l
MCV	95 fl
ESR	11 mm/h
Na	134 mmol/l
K	4.4 mmol/l
Urea	8 mmol/l
Creatinine	110 μmol/l
Albumin	36 g/l
Globulin	22 g/l
Bilirubin	11 μmol/l
ALP	1014 U/l
ALT	16 U/l
Corrected calcium	2.39 mmol/l
TSH	2.1 mU/l

Question

What is the most likely diagnosis?

Answer

This elderly man has Paget's disease of the skull causing deafness and headaches. Other complications include: fractures, sarcoma, gout, high output cardiac failure, hypercalcaemia, and platybasia (compression of the brainstem from Paget's disease at the base of the skull). Paget's disease is common in the elderly and affects 10% of people over the age of 85 years.

Paget's Disease

In Paget's disease there is increased resorption of bone and its replacement by abnormal new bone that has a thickened texture or sclerotic appearance radiologically. The bones of the axial skeleton are preferentially involved: skull, spine, pelvis, sacrum and femora. This chaotic remodelling leads to bowing of the long bones in the legs and increased risk of fractures. The increased vascularity may rarely produce cardiac failure. Deafness is due to disease of the bones in the auditory chain, or bony encasement of the cochlea and eighth nerve. Optic atrophy is also possible. The risk of sarcoma is rare (1% of patients) and is suggested by increased bone pain and the appearance of lytic lesions. The serum calcium and phosphate are normal, but hypercalcaemia with renal stones can complicate immobilisation such as following a fracture. The very high ALP is typical and urinary hydroxyproline is elevated, both reflect increased bone turnover. The treatment is simple analgesia and measures to reduce bone resorption such as: calcitonin (s/c or IM) and bisphosphonates (risedronate or etidronate by mouth and pamidronate IV). Courses of bisphosphate treatment can be given every 3 months and lead to a reduction in bone pain and fall in alkaline phosphatase.

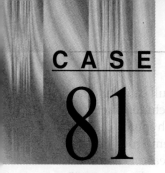

C A S E
81

CASE 81

A 69-year-old man was admitted to hospital for recurrent falls and behavioural problems, including aggressiveness and wandering. Dementia was diagnosed 3 years ago and in the last 6 months his wife found it increasing difficult to provide for his daily care. He had become verbally aggressive and accused her of having affairs with other men. He was convinced that his parents, who had died many years ago, were still living in the same house. Although he had retired more than 10 years ago, he tried repeatedly to get to work even in the small hours of the morning. On admission, he refused to take tablets, because he believed they were poisoned. Haloperidol 2 mg tds was given IM. Over the next five days he became more co-operative and agreed to take thioridazine 25 mg bd orally. One morning on returning from the toilet he fell and landed on his left hip. X-rays showed no bony injuries. The next day he refused to get out of bed, verbally abused the nursing staff, and tried to bite all those who came nearby. Paracetamol was prescribed for his pain, the dose of thioridazine was increased to 50 mg bd, additional doses of IM haloperidol given. He became febrile and trimethoprim was started for a possible urinary tract infection. He then became drowsy with slurred speech and doubly incontinent. It was impossible to administer fluids or food by mouth. The medical registrar was asked to review the patient. On examination, there were many bruises around the head, trunk and limbs. The patient's temperature was 41° Celsius, pulse 110 bpm, BP 110/80mmHg, and respiratory rate 36 per minute. There were coarse crackles in both lung bases. The heart sounds and abdomen were normal. The patient's head, neck, and limbs were rigid and could not be induced to relax. The following investigations were obtained:

Hb	14.6 g/dl
WBC	21.8 x 10⁹/l (90% Neutrophils)
Platelets	247 x 10⁹/l
CRP	82 mg/l
Na	152 mmol/l
K	3.3 mmol/l
Urea	49 mmol/l
Creatinine	209 µmol/l
Glucose	7.1 mmol/l
Albumin	39 g/l
Globulin	31 g/l
Bilirubin	13 µmol/l
ALT	63 U/l
ALP	146 U/l
Corrected calcium	2.3 mmol/l
PO₄	1.5 mmol/l
CK	2641 U/l
Urinalysis	1+ blood and 1+ protein (catheter urine specimen)
CXR	consolidation both lower lobes
ECG	sinus tachycardia

Questions
1. What are the possible clinical diagnoses?
2. What further tests are needed?
3. What is the treatment?

Answers

The possible clinical diagnoses are:

1. Hypernatraemia and uraemia due to water loss from pyrexia and poor oral fluid intake.
2. Sepsis (chest infection and urinary tract infection)
3. Subdural haematoma
4. Muscle trauma from recent falls and repeated intramuscular injections
5. Neuroleptic malignant syndrome or neuroleptic induced parkinsonism

The following tests would help:
- Blood and urine cultures
- Arterial blood gases
- CT brain
- Urinary myoglobin

The following treatment would be needed:
- IV fluids: 5% dextrose initially
- Consider CVP to guide fluid management
- Bladder catheter and measure hourly urine volumes
- Tepid sponging, antipyretics, and cooling fan for pyrexia
- Broad spectrum IV antibiotic
- Stop neuroleptic. Give benzodiazepine for agitation.
- Dantrolene

The presence of a high CK, fever and muscular rigidity should alert the clinician to the possibility of neuroleptic malignant syndrome (NMS), which is a rare complication of neuroleptic therapy. The neck stiffness could be part of the generalised muscular rigidity, rather than meningitis. In obtunded patients, who may have raised intracranial pressure, the possible risks of LP may outweigh any diagnostic advantages. While waiting for bacteriological evaluations, the initial antibiotic regime for these sick patients will need to cover the possibility of meningitis and septicaemia. The British National Formulary (*www.bnf.org.uk*) gives guidance on initial 'blind' therapy for suspected meningitis and septicaemia:

Initial 'blind' therapy for meningitis
- benzylpenicillin
- *or* cefotaxime

Initial 'blind' therapy for septicaemia
- aminoglycoside + broad spectrum penicillin
- *or* cefotaxime (alternatively ceftazidime) alone
- *or* imipenem alone

The choice depends on local resistance patterns and clinical presentation: use aminoglycoside + broad spectrum penicillin if pseudomonas suspected; add metronidazole if anaerobic infection is suspected; add flucloxacillin or vancomycin if Gram-positive infection suspected.

Neuroleptic Malignant Syndrome
- The incidence of NMS is approximately 0.1% in patients taking neuroleptics.
- 90% of patients who develop NMS will do so within 10 days of starting neuroleptic treatment. Rapid initiation, large dose escalations, and IM depots are risk factors for NMS.
- NMS occurs at any time during neuroleptic treatment, or after an increase in dosage.
- NMS can be precipitated by newer atypical antipsychotic drugs (e.g. clozapine, risperidone), although the incidence appears lower.
- NMS occurs with other drugs that block central dopamine (e.g. prochlorperazine, promethazine, metoclopramide, lithium) and in response to withdrawal of anti-parkinsonian medication.

Pathogenic Mechanism in NMS

Central mechanisms:
- Neuroleptic medications produce dopamine D2 receptor blockade.
- D2 receptor blockade in the hypothalamus impairs temperature regulation and results in hyperthermia.
- D2 receptor blockade in the nigrostriatum and extrapyramidal pathways leads to the muscular rigidity and tremor.
- D2 receptor blockade also produce sympathetic overactivity and autonomic dysfunction.

Peripheral mechanisms:
- Neuroleptics increase calcium release from sarcoplasmic reticulum, which in turn leads to increased contractility and muscle breakdown.

Diagnostic criteria for NMS

NMS is a clinical diagnosis, which is suggested by:
- Recent treatment with neuroleptics
- Hyperthermia (temperature > 38° Celsius)
- Muscular rigidity (cf. in heat stroke there is muscular flaccidity and dry skin)
- Change in mental status
- Autonomic instability (tachycardia, labile blood pressure, profuse sweating, sialorrhoea)
- Metabolic acidosis
- Elevations in CK, ALT, AST, ALP, and WBC reflect muscle damage and necrosis.
- Features of rhabdomyolysis (myoglobinuria, hyperkalaemia, hyperphosphataemia and hypocalcaemia)

Treatment of NMS
- IV fluids
- Cooling measures
- For rhabdomyolysis, urinary alkalinisation (pH > 6) with 1.4% sodium bicarbonate will promote renal excretion of myoglobin
- Beta-blockers for tachycardia
- Dopamine agonist will reverse D2 receptor blockade produced by neuroleptics. These include bromocriptine, amantadine, L-dopa, and apomorphine – all have been tried in NMS.
- Muscle relaxants: dantrolene sodium and diazepam
- Electroconvulsive therapy (ECT) for NMS has also been described, but will expose these patients to the risks of a general anaesthetic.

Prognosis of NMS
- Mortality in recent reports 10-20%, and is highest in patients with rhabdomyolysis
- NMS can recur if the same neuroleptic or a different one is introduced

Note: Thioridazine was withdrawn from the UK market in view of its propensity to cause prolonged QT syndrome.

Serotonin Syndrome (SS)

The aetiology of the serotonin syndrome is hyperstimulation of 5- HT receptors. The amino acid L-trytophan is converted to 5-hydroxytrytophan (5-HT or serotonin) and stored inside neuronal vesicles. 5-HT is then metabolised by monoamine oxidase (MAO) to 5-hydroxyindoleacetic acid. MAO-A has a greater affinity for 5-HT and, therefore, MAO-A inhibitors have a greater propensity for causing the serotonin syndrome.

Drugs causing serotonin syndrome	Proposed mechanisms
Selective serotonin reuptake inhibitor (SSRI) Tricyclic antidepressant, MDMA* Dextromethorphan, St. John's wort	Prevents 5-HT uptake
Monoamine oxidase inhibitor (MAOI) Amfetamines, MDMA*, cocaine, fenfluramine	Prevents metabolism of stored 5-HT Increased release of stored 5-HT
Buspirone, lysergic acid diethylamide (LSD)	Direct stimulation of 5-HT receptors
L-tryptophan	Increased precursor availability
Lithium	Unknown mechanism

Notes:
- *MDMA or Ecstasy is an amfetamine derivative called 3,4-methylenedioxymethamfetamine.
- Serotonin syndrome may occur when a second serotoninergic agent is inadvertently taken, including over the counter cold cures containing dextromethorphan or herbal remedies such as St. John's wort.
- Serotonin syndrome can occur with drug interactions, including failure to observe an adequate washout period between agents, e.g. between SSRI and MAOI.

Diagnostic Criteria for Serotonin Syndrome

The diagnosis of the serotonin syndrome is predominantly a clinical one, because there are no pathognomonic features, and requires all three of the following criteria:
1. Typical clinical manifestations:
    - Altered mental status: confusion, agitation, coma
    - Autonomic dysfunction: fever or hyperpyrexia, sweating, tachycardia, tachypnoea, hypertension

- Neuromuscular abnormalities: myoclonic jerks, hyper-reflexia, muscular rigidity, tremor
2. Recent exposure to medication that produces serotonin (5-HT) excess.
3. The absence of:
- Recent introduction of neuroleptic medication or an increase in its dosage.
- Other possible causes, such as infective, metabolic, or substance abuse.

Clearly, the most important differential diagnosis is neuroleptic malignant syndrome. Both conditions have many similarities and some important differences, which are summarised in the Table.

Comparisons between Serotonin Syndrome (SS) & Neuroleptic Malignant Syndrome (NMS)

	SS	NMS
Clinical features:		
- autonomic dysfunction	yes	yes
- altered mental status	yes	yes
- muscle rigidity	yes	yes
- hyperthermia	yes	yes
- tremor	yes	yes
- bradykinesia	no	yes
- hyperkinesias	yes	no
Mode of onset:	rapid (hours/days)	slow (days/weeks)
Offending medication:	serotoninergic	neuroleptic
Complications:		
- rhabdomyolysis	yes	yes
- renal failure	yes	yes
- DIC	yes	yes

Treatment of Serotonin Syndrome (SS)

- Stop the serotoninergic medication
- ITU and supportive care: cooling, fluids, and monitoring as described for the neuroleptic malignant syndrome
- Benzodiazepine is used as a muscle relaxant
- Serotonin antagonist: cyproheptadine, methysergide, propanolol
- Bromocriptine, which is useful in NMS, can precipitate SS and is therefore contraindicated

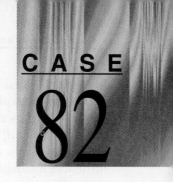

CASE 82

A 34-year-old solicitor and his wife were both ill with influenza. They rested in bed and took paracetamol for muscular pains and fever. He got up next morning, felt immediately lightheaded, and then slumped to the bedroom floor. According to the wife, he looked pale, sweated profusely, and after a few seconds opened his eyes. His speech was coherent and not confused. There was no incontinence or tongue biting. There was no past medical history and he was not taking any regular medications. An ambulance brought the patient and his wife to the A&E department. On examination, his pulse was 80 bpm, BP supine and standing 120/70 mmHg, temperature 37° Celsius. Physical examination was normal. His blood count, serum electrolytes, random blood sugar, liver function tests were all normal. ECG was unremarkable. Before the patient left the A&E department, he asked whether it would be safe for him to drive.

Question

How would you advise him?

Answer

Individuals who have suffered from a *single* episode of apparently inexplicable loss of consciousness – described in common parlance as 'lightheadedness', 'fainting', or 'blacking out' - can be a difficult diagnostic dilemma and pose awkward medicolegal concerns about their fitness to drive. There is often no history available from a reliable witness. However, headache and confusion suggest loss of consciousness from a seizure, although a single episode gives no diagnostic information on whether it is epilepsy, which is defined as 'continued tendency to have seizures'. The following is an aide-mémoire on the key points in the clinical assessment of these patients.

1. Full history is needed, including details of:
   - Prodromal symptoms*
   - Provocational factors*
   - Postural features* – whether occurring sitting or lying, or standing
   - Length of time unconscious
   - Degree of amnesia
   - Markers of seizure activity – tongue biting, incontinence, confused behaviour on recovery, headache post attack
   - * = referred to as the 3 'Ps'
2. Full physical examination, record:
   - Clinical evidence of structural heart disease
   - ECG abnormalities
   - Details of physical injury
   - You have told the patient of the obligation to inform the DVLA
   - Remind the patient that some forms of loss of consciousness are associated with a ban from driving (see below)

The Drivers and Vehicle Licensing Authority (DVLA) in the UK has provided guidance on loss of consciousness, which can be downloaded from its website: www.dvla.gov.uk. The 5 categories are summarised here.

1. Simple Faint

- Definite prevocational factors
- Prodromal symptoms
- Postural - unlikely to occur while sitting or lying

- No driving restriction applies for Group 1 (private motor cars) or Group 2 (heavy goods vehicles and public service vehicles)
- *If more than one episode, or recurring episodes, refer for further investigations as in category 3.*

2. Loss of Consciousness and Low Risk of Recurrence

- Unexplained syncope
- No relevant abnormality on cardiac and neurological examination
- Normal ECG
- Can drive 4 weeks after the event (Group 1)
- Can drive 3 months after the event (Group 2)

3. Loss of Consciousness and High Risk of Recurrence

- Unexplained syncope
- Abnormal ECG
- Clinical evidence of structural heart disease
- Syncope causing injury, occurring at the steering wheel or while sitting or lying
- More than one episode in the previous 6 months
- Require further investigations such as 48 hour ECG monitoring, ECHO, exercise ECG and specialist opinion
- Can drive 4 weeks after event if the cause has been identified and treated. If no cause identified, then require 6 months off (Group 1).
- Can drive after 3 months if the cause has been identified and treated. If no cause identified, then licence refused/revoked for one year (Group 2).

4. Witnessed (Presumed) Loss of Consciousness with Seizure Markers

- Strong clinical suspicion of epilepsy but no definite evidence
- Unconscious for > 5 minutes
- Amnesia for > 5 minutes
- Injury
- Tongue biting
- Incontinence
- Confused behaviour

- Headache post attack
- 1 year driving ban Group 1
- 5 years driving ban Group 2

5. **Loss of Consciousness with No Clinical Pointers**

- This group will have had *appropriate neurological AND cardiac opinion and investigations, but no abnormality detected.*
- 6 months ban from driving Group 1
- 1 year driving ban Group 2

CASE 83

A 72-year-old woman had radiotherapy for Cushing's disease 22 years ago. She now presented with tiredness, poor concentration and memory. Other medical problems included hypertension, hypercholesterolaemia, and diet controlled type 2 diabetes. Her medications were thyroxine 125 µg od, aspirin 75 mg od, lisinopril 2.5 mg od, and atorvastatin 40 mg od.

Hb	13.9 g/dl	
WBC	$7.2 \times 10^9/l$	
Platelets	$211 \times 10^9/l$	
ESR	5 mm/h	
Na	137 mmol/l	
K	4.2 mmol/l	
Urea	4.9 mmol/l	
Creatinine	84 µmol/l	
Glucose	5.9 mmol/l	
HbA$_{1c}$	5.8%	
Bilirubin	2 µmol/l	
AST	16 U/l	
ALP	53 U/l	
Albumin	41 g/l	
Globulin	26 g/l	
Corrected calcium	2.42 mmol/l	
Plasma ACTH levels:	09.00 h	75 ng/l
	12.00 h	50 ng/l
Plasma cortisol day curve:	09.00 h	569 nmol/l
	12.00 h	330 nmol/l
	15.00 h	344 nmol/l
	18.00 h	367 nmol/l
	21.00 h	179 nmol/l
LH	4.2 U/l	
FSH	13.4 U/l	
Prolactin	475 mU/l	

TSH	2.9 mU/l
Free T4	14.9 pmol/l
IGF-1	121 ng/ml
	(age reference = 108-229)
Glucagon stimulation test:	peak GH level = 2.3 mU/l
MRI brain	empty pituitary fossa

Question

What is the cause of her symptoms?

Answer

This patient has developed growth hormone deficiency many years after pituitary radiotherapy for Cushing's disease. The cortisol and ACTH profiles were normal, indicating no recurrence of her original hypercortisolaemia. Her diabetes was well controlled as shown by a glycated haemoglobin (HbA_{1c}) of 5.8%. The gonadotrophins (LH, FSH) were very low for a post-menopausal woman. Peak GH level in response to glucagon stimulation was very low and consistent with GH deficiency.

Adult Growth Hormone Deficiency

Growth hormone or somatropin is produced by the anterior pituitary gland. GH deficiency in adults has an estimated prevalence of 1 in 10,000 of the population. GH deficiency in children leads to dwarfism, but deficiency in adults produces subtle changes in well-being and mood, as well as a large numbers of metabolic effects.

Effects of Adult GH Deficiency

- Tiredness and impaired exercise tolerance
- Loss of muscle mass and strength
- Impaired cardiac function
- Depression and impaired libido
- Abdominal obesity
- Osteopenia or osteoporosis and a rise in fracture risk
- Increased total cholesterol and LDL cholesterol, fall in HDL
- Altered insulin sensitivity and impaired glucose tolerance
- Increased atherosclerosis risk

Causes of Adult GH Deficiency

- Pituitary tumour
- After surgery or radiotherapy for pituitary tumour
- Head trauma
- Rare infiltrative disease: sarcoidosis, tuberculosis, haemochromatosis, lymphocytic hypophysitis

Diagnosis of Adult GH Deficiency

- Peak GH levels < 9 mU/l during the hypoglycaemia of an Insulin Tolerance Test (ITT)

- Or, peak GH levels < 9 mU/l during Glucagon Stimulation Test in those patients for whom an ITT is unsafe
- Random GH levels are not useful in diagnosis
- IGF-1 may be low or normal
- In the obese or elderly, there is reduced GH production. Additional evidence of structural pituitary disease or anterior pituitary hormone deficiencies is helpful in these patients

Treatment of Adult GH Deficiency

Treatment is recommended in those with biochemical evidence of GH deficiency, typical symptoms, impaired quality of life, and reduced bone density. Currently available preparations include Genotropin, Humatrope, and Norditropin. GH treatment improves well being; increases muscle mass, bone density, and HDL; reduces body fat, abdominal adiposity, and cholesterol (total and LDL).

- Starting dose is 0.8 Units per day s/c (but commence with 0.4 Units per day s/c in those with diabetes or hypertension).
- Review clinical response, including IGF-I levels and side effects.
- Side effects include fluid retention, which presents as limb oedema, joint pain or muscle pains, carpal tunnel syndrome, rise in blood pressure, and rarely raised intracranial hypertension (suggested by the onset of headache and papilloedema). Glucose intolerance may appear in those without diabetes and diabetic control may deteriorate during GH treatment. Diabetic retinopathy needs to be monitored.
- GH replacement is contraindicated if there is active intracranial tumour.

CASE 84

This 77-year-old woman lives alone and is housebound.

Hb	10.1 g/dl
WBC	5.5 x 10⁹/l
Platelets	370 x 10⁹/l
MCV	93.1 fl
CRP	< 8 mg/l
Na	142 mmol/l
K	4.2 mmol/l
Urea	5.9 mmol/l
Creatinine	84 µmol/l
Bilirubin	5 µmol/l
ALP	132 U/l
ALT	5 U/l
Albumin	39 g/l
Globulin	35 g/l
Corrected calcium	2.1 mmol/l
PTH	15.8 pmol/l (ref 1.6-6.9)
PO₄	1.1 mmol/l

Questions

What is the diagnosis?
What test would clinch the diagnosis?

Answer

This patient has vitamin D deficiency due to chronic poor diet and lack of sunlight exposure. Her painful symptoms and leg weakness suggest osteomalacia. The normal CRP and globulins suggest that there is no sinister cause for these symptoms such as malignancy. The diagnostic test would be the 25(OH) vitamin D level, which was very low at 9 nmol/l (ref 20-110). The elevated PTH in this patient indicates secondary hyperparathyroidism, which lowers the plasma phosphate. Vitamin replacement in the form of calciferol (800 unit od) will alleviate the painful symptoms and proximal myopathy. However, the elevated alkaline phosphatase will take longer to normalize, as it depends on the healing of osteomalacic bones. Calcium levels will need to be monitored carefully and dose of calciferol adjusted as hypercalcaemia can occur.

Causes of Vitamin D deficiency

- Poor diet (e.g. vegans)
- Lack of exposure to sunlight (e.g. the elderly housebound)
- Malabsorption syndromes (e.g. pancreatic disease)
- Drugs that induce enzymes involved in vitamin D metabolism (e.g. phenytoin)

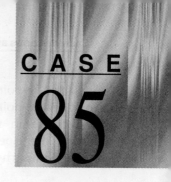

C A S E

85

CASE 85

A 65-year-old man was admitted to the CCU with an acute myocardial infarct. He received thrombolysis and on the second day felt dizzy and the ECG tracing was grossly abnormal.

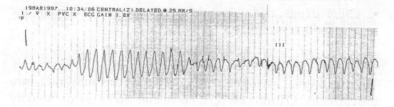

19MAR1997   10:34:06 CENTRAL(Z) DELAYED @ 25 MM/S
I / V   X   PVC X   ECG GAIN 3.0X

Question

What is the diagnosis?

Answer

Torsades-de-pointes tachycardia

Torsades-de-pointes tachycardia is a polymorphic ventricular tachycardia in which the QRS complex appears to twist around the isoelectric line. The QT interval is prolonged during sinus rhythm and there is a polymorphic U wave.

Causes of Torsades-de-pointes Tachycardia

- Bradycardia due to sick sinus syndrome or atrioventricular (AV) block.
- Antiarrhythmics
- Hypokalaemia
- Hypomagnesaemia
- Other drugs: tricyclic antidepressants, erythromycin, etc
- Congenital prolonged QT interval

Causes of Prolonged QT Interval

The QT interval varies inversely with the heart rate and hence the corrected QT interval (QT_C) is calculated as QT divided by the square root of the R-R interval (Bazett's formula). The normal QT_c does not exceed 0.42 seconds. Prolonged QT interval is seen in:

Congenital
1. Ward Romano syndrome: autosomal dominant type inheritance.
2. Jervell & Lange-Nielsen syndrome: autosomal recessive type inheritance associated with congenital deafness.

Acquired
1. Type 1A antiarrhythmics: quinidine, disopyramide, procainamide, phenothiazines, tricyclic antidepressants.
2. Type III antiarrhythmics: amiodarone, sotalol.
3. Hypocalcaemia
4. Intracranial bleeding, particularly subarachnoid haemorrhage.

Congenital Long QT (LQT) Syndrome

Individuals with congenital LQT syndrome are at risk of sudden cardiac death, seizures, or syncope during exercise or sleep. Congenital long QT syndromes show abnormalities in sodium or potassium ion channels in cardiac tissues, which are due to inherited genes. At present 6 genetic mutations are described in the Romano Ward syndrome (LQT 1 to 6) and 2 mutations in the Jervall and Lange-Nielsen syndrome (JLN 1 and 2).

Romano Ward syndrome

Genotype	Gene	Chromosome
LQT1	KVLQT1 K channel	11
LQT2	HERG K channel	7
LQT3	SCN5A Na channel	3
LQT4	Unknown gene ? ion channel	4
LQT5	CCNE1 K channel	21
LQT6	MiRP1 K channel	21

Jervall and Lange-Nielsen Syndrome

Genotype	Gene	Chromosome
JLN1	KVLQT1 K channel	11
JLN2	KCNE1 K channel	21

Management of Torsades de Pointes Tachycardia

The management of ventricular tachycardia with a polymorphic pattern depends on whether or not it occurs in the setting of a prolonged QT interval. Class IA, Class IB, and Class III drugs further prolong the QT interval and worsen the tachycardia. Therapeutic strategies should include:

- Correction of electrolyte disturbances
- Intravenous magnesium should be tried until the patient is paced
- Stop all drugs that prolong QT interval
- Atrial or ventricular temporary pacing suppresses the ventricular tachycardia, which may not recur after discontinuation of pacing

- Intravenous isoprenaline may be effective if the prolonged QT interval is acquired, but it is contraindicated in torsades de pointes tachycardia due to congenital QT prolongation.
- For long term management in patients with congenital prolongation of QT interval, beta blockers or left stellectomy may be effective. Congenital long QT syndrome is one of a number of inherited conditions associated with sudden cardiac death (SCD) for which a new treatment is an Implantable Cardioverter Defibrillator (ICD).

CASE 86

An 82-year-old lady is referred to the medical assessment unit with dizziness of 6 hours duration. She has been attending the cardiology clinic for one year and given medications for cardiac failure. On admission she was confused and her blood pressure was 98/56 mmHg. Her ECG is shown below.

Questions
1. What are the ECG diagnoses?
2. Outline the management

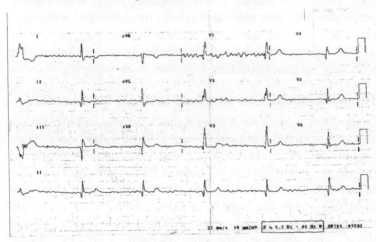

Answers

1. Complete heart block with underlying atrial fibrillation
2. The following measures are essential
- Admit the patient to the CCU
- Monitor the cardiac rhythm
- Assess the haemodynamic status: e.g. cerebral hypoperfusion (confusion) and pulmonary oedema (breathlessness)
- Prevent thromboembolic phenomena: anticoagulation if it is not contraindicated
- Review drug history, especially medications that may precipitate complete heart block such as digoxin, beta blockers, diltiazem, verapamil, etc.
- Temporary ventricular pacing is needed if the patient is symptomatic and hypotensive

This patient had no clinical or radiological evidence of cardiac failure. The old notes revealed that her atrial fibrillation had been treated with digoxin 125 µg od. Thirty years ago she had peptic ulceration with bleeding and was treated surgically. She was offered warfarin or anti-platelet therapy, but did not find the risks acceptable. After stopping the digoxin, the ventricular rate gradually increased, and on the fifth day spontaneous sinus rhythm was restored.

Thromboembolic Complications in Atrial Fibrillation

Large clinical trials have shown that warfarin and aspirin are successful in reducing the future risk of thromboembolism and stroke. The relative risk reduction in stroke produced by aspirin versus placebo is about 20%, while for warfarin versus aspirin it is 40%. In atrial fibrillation the highest risk of stroke are in the elderly (aged > 75 years, who are also more prone to bleeding complications from warfarin) and those with previous transient ischaemic attacks, stroke, diabetes, cardiac failure, and hypertension.

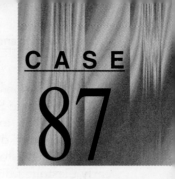

C A S E
87

CASE 87

A 68-year-old gentleman was referred to the A&E department. He had palpitations for almost two days and became dizzy in the last two hours. He smoked 20 cigarettes a day and his alcohol consumption was occasional. He had been taking ramipril 10 mg od for the past five years for hypertension. On examination, he was giddy with a blood pressure of 96/50 mmHg. There were no features of cardiac failure. An ECG was done (see below).

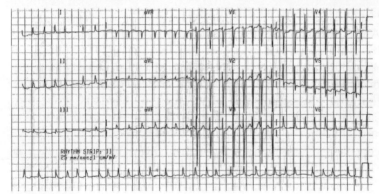

Question

What is the ECG diagnosis?

Answer

Atrial fibrillation with rapid ventricular rate in association with widespread ST segment and T wave changes. The latter could be due to rate related ischaemia or pre-existing ischaemic heart disease.

Ventricular diastolic filling occurs in three phases, namely: early diastolic filling (E), diastasis (D) and the atrial kick (A). The majority of diastolic filling occurs during the E phase which is greater than the A phase. However, the A phase still contributes to 25% of the diastolic filling of the ventricles. During atrial fibrillation, the atrial contribution to diastolic filling is lost and consequently the stroke volume and cardiac output are reduced. In the elderly, the myocardial stiffness induced by mild left ventricular hypertrophy (LVH) and other factors may lead to reversal of the E/A ratio as shown on the transmitral Doppler recording.

Diagnosis of Atrial Fibrillation

Atrial fibrillation is a supraventricular arrhythmia produced by multiple re-entrant circuits in the atria. The atrial rate is 350-600 bpm and very irregular. The atrial activity appears on the ECG as irregular fibrillary waves at rates much faster than the ventricular one. Sometimes the fibrillary waves are so fine that the atrial activity is not obvious and instead a straight line is seen between the irregularly spaced QRS complexes. Despite these high atrial rates, the atrioventricular (AV) node usually does not conduct in excess of 200 bpm. The conduction via accessory pathways can be much faster as seen in patients with atrial fibrillation and pre-excitation syndromes. The QRS complexes are narrow unless the atrial fibrillation is associated with pre-existing bundle branch block (BBB) or a rate related BBB (aberrant conduction). The QRS complexes are also wide if the atrial fibrillation results from Wolff-Parkinson-White (WPW) Syndrome.

The physical signs of atrial fibrillation include an irregularly irregular pulse, a pulse deficit between the radial pulse and apex heart rate, loss of 'a' wave in the jugular venous pulsations, and loss of the fourth heart sound. The onset of atrial fibrillation in patients with mitral stenosis, leads to the loss of presystolic accentuation in the diastolic murmur. *In clinical practice, the irregular pulse is the most important sign and it is this feature that alerts the clinician to the diagnosis of atrial fibrillation.* However, an irregular pulse can be due to atrial flutter with varying AV block or multiple extrasystoles. Multiple extrasystoles are very common in the elderly. Frequent supraventricular and ventricular extrasystolic beats (defined as > 100 beats per 24 hours) occur respectively in 26% and 14% of apparently healthy elderly people. In the elderly with cardiovascular disease, extrasystoles would be much commoner.

Chaotic (multifocal) atrial tachycardia is another cause of an irregular pulse and can only be differentiated from atrial fibrillation by an ECG. *This emphasises the importance of recording an ECG if the pulse is irregular.* Multifocal atrial tachycardia is a feature of digoxin toxicity and severe pulmonary disease especially in the elderly. It presents as an irregular narrow complex tachycardia due to several ectopic atrial foci. The ECG shows P waves that vary in axis and shape, with at least 3 differently shaped P waves (see ECG tracing below). This arrhythmia is associated with a poor prognosis as it reflects the severity of the underlying medical condition, which if treatable may abolish the arrhythmia. Digoxin is contraindicated as it worsens the arrhythmia, but verapamil may be useful.

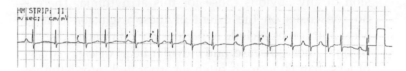

Epidemiology of Atrial Fibrillation

Atrial fibrillation occurs in 0.5% of the general population and is more common in males than females. The incidence increases steadily with advancing age. In those over 60 years of age, the incidence is 2-4% and above 75 years of age it is 11.6%. In the USA, approximately half of all patients with atrial fibrillation are older than 75 years. It is the most common cardiac arrhythmia leading to hospital admission.

Aetiology of Atrial Fibrillation

Atrial fibrillation is caused by a wide spectrum of cardiac disorders, including ischaemic heart disease, hypertension, valvular disease, cardiomyopathy, sick sinus syndrome, pericardial disease, and pre-excitation syndromes. Many extra-cardiac diseases such as infections, thyrotoxicosis, pleural disease, pulmonary thromboembolism, alcohol abuse and surgical interventions can also cause atrial fibrillation. When no aetiology is found, the condition is labelled as lone atrial fibrillation.

Lone Atrial Fibrillation

In 5-30% of all the cases of atrial fibrillation, no aetiological factor is found. The significance of lone atrial fibrillation has been subject of debate. In the Framingham study, a 2.5% rate of thromboembolism has been reported, but the mean age of these patients was 70 years and some were hypertensive or diabetic. In patients aged under 60 years with lone atrial fibrillation, only 0.55% developed thromboembolic complications after 30 years of follow up. (Kopecky SL et al. The natural history of lone atrial fibrillation. A population-based study over three decades. NEJM 1987;317:669-74).

Nowadays the term 'lone atrial fibrillation' is not generally recommended because:
- The definition of lone AF relies principally on the exclusion of any obvious cause for this arrhythmia. There is no consensus on the extent of these exclusion criteria. Most authorities exclude hypertension, pulmonary disease, coronary heart disease, and valvular heart disease. An age of less than 60 years is often incorporated into definition of lone AF.
- Some of cardiac causes of atrial fibrillation can be relatively asymptomatic and without overt physical signs such as a cardiomyopathy. *Therefore, an echocardiogram is an essential investigation in atrial fibrillation.*

Clinical Presentations of Atrial Fibrillation

Atrial fibrillation may be asymptomatic and discovered during a routine medical examination. The common symptoms include dizziness, palpitations, shortness of breath, and angina. Atrial fibrillation may be complicated by:

- Ventricular fibrillation if the ventricular rate is fast, especially in the presence of a pre-excitation syndrome such as Wolf-Parkinson-White syndrome, hypertrophic cardiomyopathy, or ischaemic heart disease.
- Tachycardiomyopathy and cardiac failure
- Thromboembolic stroke occurs in about 5% per annum in patients with non-valvular atrial fibrillation. Atrial fibrillation can be found in up to 15% of stroke patients. The risk of stroke from non-rheumatic atrial fibrillation increases with age, with a 1.5% risk of stroke in the fifth decade rising to 23.4% in the eighth decade.
- Non-valvular atrial fibrillation is associated with a five fold increase in mortality.
- Recent onset atrial fibrillation in elderly patients can have a deleterious effect on cerebral perfusion and leads to falls, confusion, and syncope.

Stratification of Atrial Fibrillation for the Risks of Stroke and Thromboembolism

(Laupacis A et al. Atrial Fibrillation Investigators. Risk Factors for Stroke and Efficacy of Antithrombotic Therapy in Atrial Fibrillation. Arch Intern Med 1994; 154: 1449-57.)

Age & Risk factor*	Stroke rate per year Placebo	Stroke rate per year Warfarin
< 65 years		
No risk factor	1%	1%
1 or more risk	4.9%	1.7%
65-75 years		
No risk factor	4.3%	1.1%
1 or more risk	5.7%	1.7%
> 75 years		
No risk factor	3.5%	1.7%
1 or more risk	8.1%	1.2%

* Risk factors for stroke are age, history of hypertension, previous transient ischaemic attack or stroke, and diabetes.

C A S E
88

CASE 88

A 28-year-old male was travelling to work when he collapsed. He was employed as a computer engineer and travelled a great deal in relation to his work. He was a non smoker and did not drink alcohol. There was no history of drug abuse. He had been fit and well prior to this collapse. There was no relevant family history. In the ambulance his capillary blood sugar was 7.4 mmol/l. Within a few hours of arriving in the casualty department he had developed a left hemiplegia and became drowsy. His blood pressure was 120/80 mmHg and pulse 80 bpm, regular in rhythm. There was no carotid bruit. He was admitted by the medical SHO and the urgent CT brain was normal. The senior medical registrar reviewed the patient and identified the signs of a right Horner's syndrome in addition to the left hemiplegia. A provisional diagnosis was made.

Questions
1. What was the provisional diagnosis?
2. What two investigations would you request to establish the diagnosis?

Answer

1. Right carotid artery dissection
2. The two diagnostic investigations are:
   - Four vessel cerebral angiography (i.e. carotid and vertebral)
   - MRI brain scan with MR angiography (MRA) of the carotid and vertebral arteries

This gentleman was referred to the local neurosurgical centre where the MRI scan confirmed ischaemic infarction in the right frontoparietal hemisphere, and the MRA showed dissection of the right internal carotid artery. He received full supportive and rehabilitative treatment along with low molecular weight heparin for 6 months. The patient made a remarkable recovery and is now living at home with minimal assistance.

Carotid and Vertebral Arterial Dissection

Ischaemic strokes in young and middle-aged patients can be secondary to arterial dissection, which may affect both the carotid and vertebral arteries. The clinical presentation depends on the artery involved and also whether it is extracranial or intracranial. The extracranial parts of these vessels are more often involved than their intracranial parts. Dissection of the carotid arteries at extracranial sites leads to anterior circulatory ischaemia (total or partial), and extracranial vertebral arterial dissection causes posterior circulatory ischaemia. The arterial wall at a dissection splits to form a false and true lumen. Blood entering the intima forms an intramural haematoma. Ischaemic stroke is the result of the true lumen being occluded by the dissection or a thrombus, or an embolism from the thrombus within the true lumen. Intracranial arterial dissection usually leads to subarachnoid haemorrhage. This is because the dissecting part of the vessel forms a pseudoaneurysm, which can then rupture.

The arterial dissection is either spontaneous or secondary to trauma. Spontaneous dissection occurs in the following conditions:

- Atheroma
- Cystic medial necrosis
- Fibromuscular dysplasia (FMD)
- Marfan's syndrome

Trauma can be penetrating or non-penetrating and relatively mild. Traumatic dissection of the internal carotid artery (ICA) is usually due to a direct blow to the neck. Dissection of the vertebral arteries is usually due to rotational and hyperextension injuries. Penetrating neck injuries tend to involve the carotids as the vertebral arteries are better protected. Dissection and intimal tears lead to an occlusive thrombus, or a non-occlusive thrombus with embolisation, resulting in a stroke within hours to weeks of the trauma. If the trauma is trivial, the patient may not recollect the original injury when he/she presents with a stroke.

Clinical Clues to Diagnosis
- History of neck trauma
- Pain in the face, around the eye, in the neck (ipsilateral to ICA dissection)
- Pain in the occiput and back of the neck (vertebral dissection)
- Horner's syndrome due to damage to the sympathetic fibres around the ICA
- Self-audible bruit
- Unilateral lower cranial nerve palsies (particularly hypoglossal) due to pressure from the expanded ICA wall at the base of the skull.

A high index of clinical suspicion is essential for diagnosis. The definitive investigation is cerebral angiography or MRA. If the carotid is completely occluded by the dissection, imaging may be nonspecific. Imaging must be done within days of symptom onset, because the dissection often resolves spontaneously.

Horner's Syndrome: Clinical Features and Aetiology
Horner's syndrome is characterised by unilateral constriction of pupil, partial ptosis and enophthalmos. There may be loss of sweating on the affected side of the face (or body), due to interruption of the sympathetic pathways. The causes of Horner's syndrome are:
1. Neurological conditions
   - Lateral medullary syndrome

- Pontine glioma
- Massive cerebral infarction
- Coning of the temporal lobe
- Syringomyelia
- Cord compression
2. Thoracic and cervical conditions
   - Cervical sympathectomy
   - Brachial plexus trauma
   - Thyroid and laryngeal surgery
   - Apical bronchogenic carcinoma
   - Cervical rib
   - Apical pulmonary tuberculosis
3. Miscellaneous
   - Congenital
   - Migrainous neuralgia
   - Idiopathic

CASE
89

CASE 89

A 60-year-old man with pruritus was treated unsuccessfully for six months by his General Practitioner and then referred to a hospital clinic. There was no anorexia, weight loss, or abdominal pain. He did not smoke and drank about 10 units of alcohol per week since his wife's death 4 years ago. He had travelled extensively, but denied any extra-marital relationships. He has never been admitted to hospital before. There was no relevant family history. Clinically he was icteric with a palpable liver. There was no lymphadenopathy or splenomegaly. The initial investigations were as follows:

Hb	12.5 g/dl
WBC	10.9 x 10⁹/l
Platelets	311 x 10⁹/l
Na	138 mmol/l
K	4.4 mmol/l
Urea	5.3 mmol/l
Creatinine	102 µmol/l
Glucose	6.2 mmol/l
Bilirubin	48 µmol/l
AST	135 U/l
ALT	195 U/l
ALP	1028 U/l
γ-GT	463 U/l
Albumin	46 g/l
Globulin	37 g/l
Hepatitis B surface antigen	not detected
Thyroglobulin antibody	negative
ANA	negative
Antismooth muscle antibody	negative
Antimitochondrial antibody	> 1280

Ultrasound and ERCP showed a normal liver with no dilatation of the intrahepatic ducts. The gall bladder and pancreas appeared normal with no gallstones. A liver biopsy showed widening of the portal tracts, non-specific inflammatory infiltration and bile duct destruction.

Question

What is the diagnosis?

Answer

Primary biliary cirrhosis

Primary Biliary Cirrhosis (PBC)

PBC predominantly affects women aged 40-50 years. The female to male ratio is six to one. The aetiology is unknown, but there is an association with other autoimmune conditions such as rheumatoid arthritis, Sjögren's syndrome, scleroderma, and the CREST syndrome (Calcinosis cutis, Raynaud's phenomenon, Esophageal motility disorder, Sclerodactyly, and Telangiectasia). Hypothyroidism due to autoimmune thyroiditis is relatively common and may eventually develop in 20% of patients with PBC. Renal tubular acidosis may also occur. There is progressive destruction of the bile ducts that leads eventually to cirrhosis. The earliest clinical presentation is pruritus, followed by jaundice months or years later. Fatigue may be a major symptom. When jaundice appears the liver is usually enlarged. Other features include hepatosplenomegaly, xanthelasma of eyelids and cholesterol deposition in palmar creases. Asymptomatic patients are discovered on routine examination, including the chance finding of unexplained hepatomegaly, an elevated ALP, or positive antimitochondrial autoantibody. The following investigations are needed:

1. Raised ALP is often the only abnormality
2. Serum IgM may be very high
3. Serum cholesterol is raised
4. Ultrasound may show diffuse alteration of the liver architecture and also exclude other causes of abnormal liver function tests.
5. Positive antimitochondrial (AMA) antibody (in titres > 1: 160) are present in 95% of cases, while the ANA and antismooth muscle antibodies may be positive or negative
6. Liver biopsy is diagnostic

Liver Biopsy in PBC

In the early stages, liver biopsy shows portal tract infiltrates of lymphocytes, plasma cells and granulomatous lesions (found in 40% of biopsies). Subsequently, there is damage and loss of the bile ducts with portal tract fibrosis and established cirrhosis. Males appear to be more likely to develop hepatocellular carcinoma. There is a group of patients with histological features of PBC, but with the serology of chronic autoimmune hepatitis i.e. positive ANA and positive antismooth muscle antibodies but negative antimitochondrial antibody. This condition has been termed autoimmune cholangitis and is responsive to steroids and azathioprine.

Differential Diagnosis of Hepatic Granulomas

- Primary biliary cirrhosis
- Sarcoidosis
- Tuberculosis
- Schistosomiasis
- Drug reactions
- Brucellosis
- Strongyloidosis

Common Causes of Liver Cirrhosis

- Alcohol
- Viral Hepatitis B, C and D (Hepatitis D occurs with B)
- Biliary cirrhosis (primary and secondary)
- Autoimmune hepatitis
- Idiopathic

Other Causes of Liver Cirrhosis

- Hereditary haemochromatosis
- Budd-Chiari syndrome
- Wilson's disease
- α1-anti-trypsin deficiency
- Cystic fibrosis
- Galactosaemia
- Glycogen storage disease
- Veno-occlusive disease

The Management of Primary Biliary Cirrhosis

Initial management is symptomatic e.g. control pruritus with antihistamines and colestyramine. Intractable pruritus may respond to rifampicin and plasmapheresis. Ursodeoxycholic acid may be beneficial in some patients leading to improvement of liver function and pruritus. Ciclosporin and colchicine have been tried in some cases. Corticosteroids and azathioprine are not helpful. Corticosteroids also aggravate osteoporosis. Associated malabsorption of vitamins A, D, and K need to be treated. Oral calcium and vitamin D are also needed for osteoporosis or osteomalacia. Hyperlipidaemia requires appropriate dietary input and colestyramine, and may be complicated by a xanthomatous polyneuropathy. Liver transplant is offered if bilirubin is > 100 mmol/l.

Differential Diagnosis of Painless Obstructive Jaundice

1. Primary biliary cirrhosis
2. Primary sclerosing cholangitis (raised ALP; negative AMA; ERCP shows multiple strictures in bile ducts; pathology is fibrotic narrowing of the bile ducts)
3. Sclerosing cholangitis is secondary to inflammatory bowel disease
4. Carcinoma of the pancreas

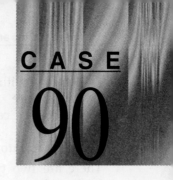

C A S E
90

CASE 90

An 82-year-old lady was admitted with a 48 hours history of breathlessness. Her past medical history included an anterior myocardial infarct 3 months ago following which her exercise tolerance had always been limited. She was tachycardic on admission with a pulse 112 beats in minute and irregular in rhythm. Her blood pressure was 100/60 mmHg. There was a gallop rhythm with jugular venous pressure at 5 cm above the sternal angle and crackles were present in both lungs. Initial oxygen saturation was low and an urgent arterial blood gas examination was obtained.

Arterial blood gases (on 2 litres of oxygen):

pH	7.44
PaO$_2$	6.22 kPa
PaCO$_2$	5.56 kPa
HCO$_3$	28.6 mmol/l
Oxygen saturation	89 %

Questions
1. What do the blood gases show?
2. What is the likely diagnosis?

Answers

1. Hypoxia with normal $PaCO_2$ suggesting a type I respiratory failure
2. Congestive cardiac failure

Type I Respiratory Failure

There are two types of respiratory failure:

1. Type I (acute hypoxaemic): a low PaO_2 with a normal or low $PaCO_2$
2. Type II (ventilatory failure): a low PaO_2 with a high $PaCO_2$

Type I respiratory failure results from damage to lung tissue and is seen in:

- Pulmonary oedema
- Pulmonary embolism
- Pneumonia
- Acute lung injury
- Fibrosing alveolitis

CASE 91

An 18-year-old university student was brought to the A&E department, because his girlfriend observed slurring of his speech and within ten minutes he could not speak. He was conscious and haemodynamically stable. The heart was in sinus rhythm and there was no clinical evidence of cardiomegaly or valvular disease. The chest and abdomen were unremarkable. He was dysphasic, but understood simple commands. The cranial nerves and optic fundi were normal. There was no evidence of motor, sensory, or cerebellar dysfunction. The carotid pulses were normal without bruits. The routine biochemical and haematological screen were normal. Blood sugar was 6 mmol/l. ECG confirmed sinus rhythm and chest X-ray was unremarkable. A CT scan of the head revealed an area of low attenuation in the left frontal lobe.

Questions

1. What are the possible causes of this young patient's acute ischaemic stroke?
2. How is this patient best managed and investigated?

Answers

In young adults with stroke consider the following:

Causes of stroke in young adults

- Ischaemic stroke   60%
- Primary intracranial haemorrhage   20%
- Subarachnoid haemorrhage   20%

Causes of ischaemic stroke in the young adults

- Athero thromboembolism (large vessel
  and small vessel disease)   30%
- Carotid dissection   20%
- Non-atherosclerosis   10%
- Haematological   5-10%
- Unknown   25%

Athero Thromboembolism

This is the commonest cause of ischaemic stroke in all ages. The usual predisposing factors are smoking, hypertension, hyperlipidaemia, and diabetes mellitus.

Cardiac Embolism

This results from a left ventricular thrombus, infective endocarditis, atrial myxoma or emboli from the right side of the heart in association with right to left shunts (atrial septal defect). The embolus usually results in a wedge shaped haemorrhagic infarct in the brain substance that is peripherally located and can involve multiple arterial distributions. Other causes are atrial myxoma and mitral valve prolapse

Non-atherosclerosis

This includes vasculitis, migraine, drug abuse, and angiitis secondary to infections (e.g. HIV, syphilis, and herpes zoster).

Haematological

Conditions such as thrombophilic states (antithrombin III, protein C and S deficiencies, factor V Leiden, antiphospholipid syndromes), and sickle cell disease.

Substance Abuse

There is a 12 fold increased incidence of stroke among drug abusers compare with non-abusers. The commonly implicated substances are cocaine, amfetamine and heroin. They cause ischaemia by inducing vasospasm, foreign body embolisation, or initiating a vasculitic process.

Dural Sinus Thrombosis

This commonly involves the superior sagittal sinus and is precipitated by conditions such as dehydration, infection, hypercoagulable states, pregnancy and the puerperium. *These infarcts are typically subcortical and haemorrhagic; the area involved does not conform to one arterial territory.* An MRI/MRA confirms the diagnosis.

2. The management and investigations of the patients with young strokes are as follows:

Acute Phase Management

- Admission to the stroke unit
- Adequate hydration
- Monitor oxygen saturation
- Maintain cerebral perfusion
- Good glycaemic control
- Temperature regulation.
- Brain imaging within 48 hours of onset, but this will be urgent if the patient shows signs suggestive of subarachnoid haemorrhage, posterior fossa signs (cerebellar dysfunction), features of increased intracranial pressure, or if they are on anticoagulants.
- Aspirin (150-300 mg) within 48 hours of the event if an ischaemic infarct is confirmed.
- Haemorrhagic stroke - refer to a neurosurgical service.
- Cerebral angiography or the less invasive magnetic resonance angiography if intracerebral bleeding, subarachnoid haemorrhage, or cervical dissection is suspected.

Investigations

- Radiological: CT scan, carotid Doppler, repeat CT and MRI scan in some patients

- Biochemical: Blood glucose, renal and liver functions, calcium, CRP (or ESR), vasculitic screen, homocysteine levels
- Haematological: thrombophilia, antiphospholipid antibodies, sickle cell disease
- Cardiac: ECG, echocardiogram (transthoracic or transoesophageal if the former cannot exclude a cardiac cause of embolisation)

Long Term Management and Secondary Stroke Prevention

One of the main principles of managing strokes is secondary prevention. This includes establishing the cause of stroke, provision of antiplatelet or anticoagulant therapy (if appropriate), and dealing with the underlying cause. Organized rehabilitation by a multidisciplinary team (doctors, physiotherapists, occupational therapists, speech therapists, psychologists, specialist stroke nurses and social workers) in specialized stroke units is an essential part of management. Patients should seek advice from The Stroke Association (*www.stroke.org.uk)*, or Different strokes (*www.differentstrokes.co.uk)* which provides practical support to young strokes.

Medical interventions for secondary prevention can be summarized as follows:

- All patients with cerebral infarctions should remain on an antiplatelet agent, e.g. aspirin. However, if there is aspirin intolerance, either dipyridamole or clopidogrel can be used. In cases of aspirin failure i.e. recurrent strokes despite aspirin therapy, one can add either dipyridamole or clopidogrel.
- Anticoagulation in patients with atrial fibrillation, mural thrombus, or a positive thrombophilia screen.
- Blood pressure maintained at the target of ≤ 140 mmHg systolic and diastolic blood pressure ≤ 85 mmHg
- Good glycaemic control in diabetic patients
- Patients with a total cholesterol concentration greater than 5 mmol/l and ischaemic stroke due to arterial disease or in the presence of previous myocardial infarction or angina, should be commenced on statin therapy
- The HOPE study has also shown that ramipril (angiotensin converting enzyme inhibitor) reduces the risk of stroke regardless of whether the patients were hypertensive or normotensive.

Prognosis of Stroke in Young Patients

In England and Wales, the annual incidence of first ever stroke is about 110,000 and an additional 30,000 patients have a recurrent stroke. Stroke is mostly prevalent in the elderly and increases with age. After the age of 55 years, for each successive 10 years, the stroke rate doubles. Many authorities define young strokes as those who are under 45 years of age and they account for about 10% of all strokes.

The annual incidence rate of young stroke is estimated at 10.23 per 100,000 (Marini et al 2001). The prognosis of stroke in young adults < 45 years was studied in a population of 297,838 individuals. In this population, 174,875 (58.7%) individuals were aged < 45 years. Over a 5 year period, there were 4,353 patients with first ever stroke, including 89 patients (= 2% of all strokes) who were aged < 45 years. The type of strokes according to age group is shown below.

Type of Stroke*	Age < 45 years		Age > 45 years	
Subarachnoid haemorrhage	22.5%		2.4%	
Intracerebral haemorrhage	20.2%	42.7%	13.3%	15.7%
Cerebral infarction	57.3%		83.1%	

(* L'Aquila Registry, Marini et al 2001)

In this study by Marini et al, young patients have a much higher prevalence of subarachnoid haemorrhage and intra-cerebral haemorrhage (42.7%) compared with the older patients (15.7%). The 30 day mortality in young stroke patients was 11% (n=10 patients): 7 patients had intracranial haemorrhage, and 3 patients had subarachnoid haemorrhage. No patient with cerebral infarction died in the first 30 days post stroke. In young patients subarachnoid haemorrhage had the highest proportion of good recovery (60%), intracerebral haemorrhage had the highest mortality (44%), and cerebral infarction had the highest proportion of severe disability (47%).

A study by Kappelle et al of 296 young patients with ischaemic stroke provided more information about mortality and recurrence rates. Twenty-one patients (7%) died as the result of their initial stroke, and another 40 patients (14%) died during a mean follow-up of 6.0 years. None of the patients aged 25 years or younger at the time of stroke died during follow-up. Mortality was significantly higher among patients who had a stroke secondary to large-vessel disease and significantly lower in patients with stroke of unknown aetiology. Recurrent strokes occurred in 23 patients (9%) and were fatal in 9 patients. The authors concluded that the risks of recurrent vascular events in young adults who have had ischaemic stroke are considerable. In addition, the majority of survivors will have residual emotional, social, or physical impairments that hamper employment or lower the quality of life.

Two other studies on young patients (< 45 years) with ischaemic strokes showed more favourable long-term outcomes (Hindfelt B & Nilsson O 1977, Hindfelt B & Nilsson O 1992). Both studies had smaller number of patients with low immediate mortality and long-term mortality, and re-infarction rates.

References
- Marini C, Totaro R, De Santis F, Ciancarelli I, Baldassarre M, Carolei A. Stroke in young adults in the community-based L'Aquila registry: incidence and prognosis. Stroke 2001 32(1):52-6.
- Kappelle LJ, Adams HP Jr, Heffner ML, Torner JC, Gomez F, Biller J. Prognosis of young adults with ischaemic stroke: A long-term follow-up study assessing recurrent vascular events and functional outcome in the Iowa Registry of Stroke in Young Adults. Stroke 1994: 25(7):1360-5.
- Hindfelt B, Nilsson O. Long-term prognosis of ischaemic stroke in young adults. Acta Neurologica Scandinavica. 1992: 86(5):440-5.
- Hindfelt B. Nilsson O. The prognosis of ischaemic stroke in young adults. Acta Neurologica Scandinavica 1997: 55(2):123-30.

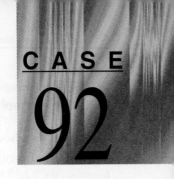
CASE 92

An 88-year-old man was referred by his General Practitioner after a routine blood test. Examination by the hospital specialist revealed mild hepatosplenomegaly. There was no lymphadenopathy. The full blood count result is given below:

Hb	11.0 g/dl
WBC	575 x 10⁹/l
Platelets	89 x 10⁹/l
Neutrophil	12.8 x 10⁹/l
Lymphocyte	568 x 10⁹/l
Monocyte	2.3 x 10⁹/l
Eosinophil	0
Basophil	0
Na	137 mmol/l
K	4.5 mmol/l
Urea	3.0 mmol/l
Creatinine	78 µmol/l
Albumin	27 g/l
Globulin	32 g/l
Bilirubin	5 µmol/l
ALP	178 U/l
ALT	7 U/l
AST	16 U/l
IgA	1.65 g/l (ref 0.7 – 4.0)
IgG	12.05 g/l (ref 5.4 – 16.5)
IgM	3.43 g/l (ref 0.5 –2)

Questions
1. What are the abnormalities?
2. What is the diagnosis?

Answers

1. Lymphocytosis with thrombocytopenia and anaemia.
2. Chronic lymphocytic leukaemia (CLL)

Chronic Lymphocytic Leukaemia (CLL)

Uncontrolled proliferation of lymphocytes is the characteristic feature of CLL. They usually are B-lymphocytes, although T-lymphocytes are also described. CLL may be asymptomatic, being diagnosed incidentally. The common clinical features include: anaemia (secondary to marrow involvement or hae-molysis), bleeding, recurrent infections, painless lymph node enlargement, and splenomegaly. About half of the patients may have constitutional symptoms such as weight loss, fever, sweating, malaise, and fatigue. Herpes zoster is a common complication. Leukaemic complications may involve the skin, lungs, mediastinal lymph nodes, brain or the kidneys and urinary tract.

Investigations

- Low or normal haemoglobin
- White cell count $> 15 \times 10^9/l$ with at least 40% of them being lymphocytes
- Low or normal platelets
- Low or normal serum immunoglobulins
- Positive Coombs' test in cases complicated by haemolysis
- Blood film: small lymphocytes (they have not matured normally and are immunologically incompetent).
- Immunophenotyping: lymphocytes co-express the CD5 and CD19 antigen

Management

The disease can remain asymptomatic for many years. Occasionally it can progress to a high grade Non-Hodgkin's lymphoma that responds poorly to treatment. There are two ways of staging CLL that correlate well with the prognosis and help in the management of this condition. These include the Rai staging system (Table 1) and the Binet staging system (Table 2). Lymphocytosis is present in all stages of the disease. Progression of the disease is defined by weight loss, fatigue, fever, massive organomegaly and a rapidly rising lymphocyte count. Lymphoid areas include cervical, inguinal and axillary lymph nodes.

Table 1: Rai Staging System

Stage	Risk of progression	Manifestations	Median survival (years)	Recommended treatment
0	Low	Lymphocytosis	> 10	Watch and wait
I	Intermediate	Lymphadenopathy	9	Treat only with progression
II	Intermediate	Splenomegaly, lymphadenopathy, or both	7	Treat only with progression
III	High	Anaemia, organomegaly, or both	5	Treatment indicated in most cases
IV	High	One or more: anaemia, organomegaly and thrombocytopenia	5	Treatment indicated in most cases

Table 2: Binet Staging System

Stage	Risk of progression	Manifestations	Median survival (years)	Recommended treatment
A	Low	< 3 lymphoid areas enlarged* Hb > 10 g/dl	> 10	Wait and see
B	Intermediate	≥ 3 lymphoid areas enlarged Platelets < 100 x 10^9/l	7	Treatment indicated in most cases
C	High	Hb < 10 g/dl Platelets < 100 x 10^9/l	5	Treatment indicated in most cases

* The neck, axilla and groin lymph node groups (whether unilateral or bilateral), liver and spleen each represent one area.

As the disease may be stable over many years, treatment is indicated only when the disease progresses with the development of anaemia, infections, bleeding or lymphadenopathy. The therapeutic agents are:

- Chlorambucil, used intermittently with prednisolone
- High dose corticosteroids for haemolytic anaemias

Causes of Lymphocytosis

Lymphocytosis is defined as a lymphocyte count > $5.0 \times 10^9/l$. Causes include:

1. Viral infections
   - Epstein-Barr virus
   - Cytomegalovirus
   - HIV
2. Chronic infections
   - Tuberculosis
   - Toxoplasmosis
3. CLL
4. Some lymphomas

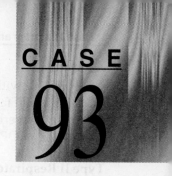

CASE 93

A 72-year-old man was admitted with progressively worsening breathlessness over the last 24 hours. He has had recurrent hospital admissions for the same problem. On examination, he was tachycardic and drowsy. There were nicotine stains on the fingers of the right hand. The chest was hyperinflated with a barrel shaped configuration and widespread wheezes could be heard in both lungs. His oxygen saturation was low and an arterial blood gas examination was performed urgently.

Arterial blood gases (on 2 litres of oxygen):

pH	7.27
PaO_2	7.15 kPa
$PaCO_2$	8.17 kPa
HCO_3	27.9 mmol/l
Oxygen saturation	85 %

Questions
1. What do the blood gases show?
2. What is the likely diagnosis?

Answers

1. Hypoxia with hypercapnia consistent with type II respiratory failure
2. Acute exacerbation of Chronic Obstructive Pulmonary Disease (COPD)

Type II Respiratory Failure

Respiratory failure is present when $PaO_2 < 8.0$ kPa (60 mmHg) or the $PaCO_2$ is > 7 kPa (55 mmHg). There are two types of respiratory failure:

Type I: a low PaO_2 with a normal or low $PaCO_2$

Type II: a low PaO_2 with a high $PaCO_2$

Type II respiratory failure results from inadequate alveolar ventilation, such as in:

- COPD (the commonest cause)
- Chest wall abnormalities
- Respiratory muscle weakness (Guillain-Barré syndrome)
- Depression of respiratory centre (e.g. opiate drugs)

The British Thoracic Society Guidelines on Diagnosis and Treatment of Acute Exacerbation of COPD [The COPD Guidelines Group of the Standards of Care Committee of the BTS. BTS Guidelines for the Management of Chronic Obstructive Pulmonary Disease. Thorax 1997: 52 (Suppl 5); S1-S25]

Definition of COPD

a. Chronic obstructive pulmonary disease (COPD) is a general term which covers many previously used clinical labels that are now recognised as being different aspects of the same problem.

b. Diagnostic labels encompassed by COPD include:
   - Chronic bronchitis
   - Emphysema
   - Chronic obstructive airways disease
   - Chronic airflow limitation
   - Some cases of chronic asthma.

c. COPD is a chronic, slowly progressive disorder characterised by airways obstruction ($FEV_1 < 80\%$ predicted and FEV_1/VC ratio $< 70\%$), which does not change markedly over several months. The impairment of lung function is largely fixed but is partially reversible by bronchodilator (or other) therapy.

d. Most cases are caused by tobacco smoking.

e. COPD causes significantly more mortality and morbidity than do other causes of airflow limitation in adults.

Diagnosis of COPD

a. The diagnosis is usually suggested by symptoms (see below) but can only be established by objective measurement, preferably using spirometric tests.

b. Unlike asthma, airflow limitation in COPD as measured by the FEV_1 can never be returned to normal values. However, treatment can improve both symptoms and measured airflow limitation.

c. The symptoms and signs vary with the severity of the disease.

Category	FEV_1 (% predicted)	Symptoms and signs of COPD
Mild	60-80	No abnormal signs. Smoker's cough. Little or no breathlessness.
Moderate	40-59	Breathlessness (± wheeze) on moderate exertion. Cough (± sputum). Variable abnormal signs (general reduction in breath sounds, presence of wheezes).
Severe	< 40	Breathlessness on any exertion/at rest. Wheeze and cough often prominent. Lung over inflation usual; cyanosis, peripheral oedema and polycythaemia in advanced disease, especially during exacerbations.

Presenting Features of Acute Exacerbations of COPD

• Worsening of previous stable condition
• Increased wheeze
• Increased dyspnoea
• Increased sputum volume
• Increased sputum purulence
• Chest tightness
• Fluid retention

Home Treatment of Acute Exacerbations

a. Add or increase bronchodilators (consider if inhaler device and technique are appropriate).

b. Prescribe an antibiotic if two or more of the following are present:
   - Increased breathlessness
   - Increased sputum volume
   - Development of purulent sputum

c. Oral corticosteroids may be prescribed in some cases. These should not be used unless:
   - The patient is already on oral corticosteroids
   - There is a previously documented response to oral corticosteroids
- Airflow obstruction fails to respond to an increase in bronchodilator dosage
- This is the first presentation of airflow obstruction

Hospital Treatment of Acute Exacerbation

a. Hospital treatment of an acute exacerbation is as for home treatment except:

Drug	Criteria	Action
Bronchodilator	Moderate exacerbation	Nebulised β_2 agonist or ipratropium bromide. If no response, consider IV aminophylline.
	Severe exacerbation	Nebulised ipratropium bromide and β_2 agonist in combination. If no response, consider IV aminophylline.
Oxygen	Moderate/Severe exacerbation	Given in ambulance or on arrival, 24-28% mask 2 litres/min by nasal prongs. Check blood gases within 60 minutes of starting oxygen, modify flow rate according to PaO_2 and pH.

b. If pH is < 7.26 and $PaCO_2$ is rising consider ventilatory support. This may be by intubation and intermittent positive pressure ventilation (IPPV) or non-invasive IPPV, although the latter is probably best initiated at a higher pH and is only suitable in cooperative patients without excessive secretions. An alternative is the use of intravenous doxapram.

c. IPPV is likely to be appropriate when:
- There is a clear basis for the current deterioration
- It is the first episode of respiratory failure
- There is an acceptable quality of life/habitual level of activity
- The patient has not previously had a full medical assessment
- There are few if any co-morbidity

d. A senior doctor must make the decision not to institute ventilatory support.

e. Neither age nor the $PaCO_2$ predict survival.

Follow Up of Acute Exacerbations

Follow up assessment 4-6 weeks after discharge from hospital should include:
- Patient's ability to cope
- Measurement of FEV_1
- Reassessment of inhaler technique and patient's understanding of recommended treatment regime
- Need for long term oxygen therapy (LTOT) and home nebuliser usage in patients with severe COPD
- Follow up thereafter is as for stable COPD.

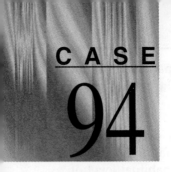

CASE

94

CASE 94

A 45-year-old woman was referred to the hospital clinic with a 4 months history of exertional breathlessness. She was a non-smoker and has been well prior to this illness. Her brother aged 50 years has hypertension and diabetes. General physical examination was unremarkable. There were no cardiac murmurs and the lungs were clear. Her blood pressure was 190/90 mmHg and pulse 60 bpm regular. Urinalysis, haematology, biochemistry, and chest X-ray were all normal. The ECG and echocardiogram both showed evidence of left ventricular hypertrophy. An ambulatory blood pressure (ABP) was obtained and displayed below:

Summary over 24 hours

	Min	Mean	Max	SD
Systolic (mmHg)	138	171	228	18.20
Diastolic (mmHg)	69	86	111	9.19
MAP (mmHg)	97	119	147	12.11
Heart Rate (bpm)	55	65	74	4.08

Percent of Systolic Readings above period limits: 96.7 %
Percent of Diastolic Readings above period limits: 43.3 %
Percent of time Systolic was above period limits: 97.1 %
Key: SD = standard deviation
         bpm = beats per minute
         MAP = mean arterial pressure

Summary: 06:00 to 21:00 hours

	Min	Mean	Max	SD
Systolic (mmHg)	138	170	228	19.42
Diastolic (mmHg)	69	86	111	10.11
MAP (mmHg)	97	119	147	13.20
Heart Rate (bpm)	55	64	74	3.93

Percent of Systolic Readings > 140 mmHg: 95.6 %
Percent of Diastolic Readings > 85 mmHg: 40.0 %
Percent of time Systolic > 140 mmHg: 95.8 %
Percent of time Diastolic > 85 mmHg: 38.9 %

Summary: 21:00 to 06:00 hours

	Min	Mean	Max	SD
Systolic (mmHg)	146	176	205	13.10
Diastolic (mmHg)	80	88	100	5.71
MAP (mmHg)	106	120	139	8.28
Heart Rate (bpm)	61	67	70	2.97

Percent of Systolic Readings > 140 mmHg: 100.0 %
Percent of Diastolic Readings > 85 mmHg: 53.3 %
Percent of time Systolic > 140 mmHg: 100.0 %
Percent of time Diastolic > 85 mmHg: 49.6 %

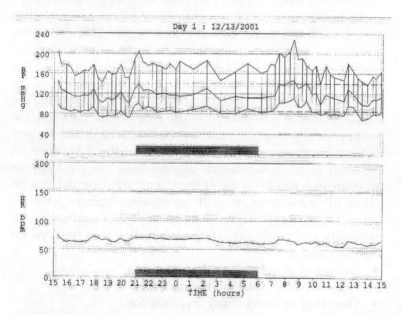

Question
What does the ABP recording show?

Answer

The ABPM shows poorly controlled hypertension with a non-dipping pattern at night-time.

Circadian Rhythm in Blood Pressure

In people who are healthy, circadian rhythm in blood pressure is well established, with a 10% to 20% decrease in systolic and diastolic blood pressure during night-time. This is described as nocturnal 'dipping' of blood pressure. People whose blood pressure does not dip at night-time are called 'non-dippers'. It has been shown that non-dipping of blood pressure at night-time is associated with end organ damage.

Ambulatory Blood Pressure Monitoring (ABPM)

Ambulatory blood pressure monitoring uses portable equipment to obtain multiple recordings of blood pressure (BP) measurements during the day and night. This technique produces a profile showing the variation in the BP readings during the course of a 24 hour period. Setting up an ABPM service and selecting the monitor have been described by O'Brien et al 2000. Various devices for ABPM monitoring are available, but it is important to use a device that is validated independently according to the protocol of the British Hypertension Society, or the US Association for the Advancement of Medical Instrumentation. Studies have shown that the daytime average BP is lower than clinic BP. Compared with clinic BP measurements, ABP profiles are a more sensitive predictor of target organ damage and also cardiovascular mortality and morbidity. The possible clinical indications for ABPM include:

- Exclusion of white coat hypertension
- Hypertension resistant to treatment
- Detection of ambulatory hypotension
- Deciding on treatment in borderline hypertension
- Identification of nocturnal hypertension
- Hypertension in pregnancy
- As a guide to treatment in elderly people with hypertension (see below)

Ambulatory BP in Elderly Patients

A variety of ambulatory of blood pressure patterns have been observed in the elderly, which include the following:

- White coat hypertension
- Isolated systolic hypertension
- Postural hypotension
- Post-prandial hypotension
- Daytime hypotension/nocturnal hypertension
- Drug induced hypotension
- Autonomic failure

Isolated systolic hypertension is very common in the elderly. The SYST-Eur Trial (Staessen et al 1999) showed that the systolic BP measured conventionally may average 20 mmHg higher than the day time ambulatory BP levels. Therefore, conventional methods may significantly over diagnose isolated systolic hypertension in the elderly and subject these patients to unnecessary treatments. Furthermore, elderly patients commonly show side effects of BP medications, such as hypotensive episodes, which can bedemonstrated on ABPM.

Indications for ABPM

The British Hypertension Society (Ramsay LE et al. British Hypertension Society guidelines for hypertension management 1999: summary. BMJ 1999; 319: 630-35) has suggested the following clinical indications for ABP measurement:

- Diagnosis of white coat hypertension
- Hypertension that is resistant to drug treatment [> 3 drugs]
- When BP readings in the clinic show unusual variability
- When hypotension is suspected

ABPM Reference Values

Based on a number of different studies the following recommendations have been made on the normal and abnormal levels in ABPM readings (O'Brien et al 2000):

	Normal	Abnormal
Day	≤ 135/85	>140/90
Night	≤ 120/70	>125/75
24 hour	≤ 130/80	>135/85

Fitting the Monitor

The monitor is initialised with patient details. The BP is measured in both arms and if the difference is < 10 mmHg, then the non-dominant arm is used. If difference is > 10 mmHg, then the arm with higher pressure is used. The cuff size should be appropriate and the frequency of measurement should be selected as follows:

	Dimension of the sphygmomanometer cuff
Child or lean adult	12 cm × 18 cm
Adult	12 cm × 26 cm
Adult with large arm	12 cm × 40 cm

Preparing the Patient

- Explaining the test: reason for ABPM, frequency of blood pressure recording.
- Instructions: the patient should rest the arm at heart level during recordings; inactivate the monitor after 24 hours; manually deflate cuff if the need arises.
- Provide the patient with contact details of the doctor or team if any need arises, and give a diary card to record any symptoms.

Analysing the Data

- Number of measurements needed:
  Day: >14 Systolic and Diastolic BP
  Night: > 7 Systolic and Diastolic BP
- Mean day time Systolic and Diastolic BP
- Mean night time Systolic and Diastolic BP
- Mean 24 hour Systolic and Diastolic BP

Disadvantage and Causes of Poor Data

- Inconvenience to patients.
- Poor technique
- Arrhythmias
- Small pulse volume
- Device failure

References

- O'Brien E, Beevers G, Lip GYH. ABC of Hypertension; Blood pressure measurement: Part III- Automated sphygmomanometry: ambulatory blood pressure measurement. BM J 2001: 322; 1110-14.
- O'Brien E, Coates A, Owens P, Petrie J, Padfield PL, Littler WA, de Swiet M, Mee F. Use and interpretation of ambulatory blood pressure monitoring: recommendations of the British Hypertension Society. BMJ 2000: 320; 1128-34.
- Owens P and O'Brien ET. Hypotension: a forgotten illness? Blood Press Monitoring 1997;2:3-14.
- Staessen J, Thijs L, Fagard R, for the Systolic Hypertension in Europe (SYST-Eur) Trial Investigators. Conventional and ambulatory blood pressure as predictors of cardiovascular risk in older patients with systolic hypertension. J Hypertens 1999; 17(Suppl 3):S16.

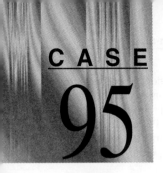

C A S E
95

CASE 95

A 48-year-old man presented with blurring of vision in the right eye. Examination of the right fundus showed changes compatible with central retinal vein thrombosis. There was a large abdominal mass extending from the left hypochondrium to the left iliac fossa. It was dull on percussion and the examining hand could not get above it. There was no evidence of lymphadenopathy or hepatomegaly. The medical registrar arranged for an urgent full blood count and blood film. The results were as follows:

Hb	8.2 g/dl
WBC	298 x 10^9/l
Platelets	468 x 10^9/l
ESR	10 mm/h
MCV	99 fl
MCH	31.2 pg
MCHC	32.2 g/dl

Differential WBC Count

Neutrophils	48%
Lymphocytes	2%
Monocytes	1%
Eosinophils	1%
Metamyelocytes	8%
Myelocytes	20%
Promyelocytes	4%
Blast cells	16%

Blood film reported the followings: anisocytosis, polychromasia, myeloblasts and nucleated red cells.

Questions
1. What is the most likely diagnosis?
2. What diagnostic test is required?
3. Name two other investigations that may be useful

Answers
1. Chronic myeloid leukaemia
2. Bone marrow aspirate
3. Two other useful investigations are Philadelphia chromosome and leucocyte alkaline phosphatase

Philadelphia Chromosome (Ph¹)

About 95% of patients with CML show the Philadelphia chromosomal abnormality. The Philadelphia chromosome is produced by a reciprocal translocation between chromosome 9 and chromosome 22: t(9;22). See figure below.

- The long arm of chromosome 9 breaks near the *abl* proto-oncogene region.
- The long arm of chromosome 22 breaks near the middle of a gene called *bcr* ('break point cluster').
- Most of the long arm of 22 is relocated to 9. This results in a longer chromosome 9 [9q+].
- The *abl* region from 9 is then relocated to the truncated long arm of 22 near its *bcr* region.
- The *bcr-abl* fusion gene on the Philadelphia chromosome [22q- (Ph¹)] encodes for a chimeric protein that has tyrosine kinase activity (i.e. attaches phosphate groups to proteins) and ultimately leads to unrestrained cellular proliferation and protection from apoptosis (cell death).
- Another mutation later occurs in these Philadelphia chromosome bearing cells, rendering them unable to differentiate properly and a blast crisis phase ensues.
- Imatinib mesylate (Glivec) inhibits cellular proliferation and induces apoptosis and shows promise in the treatment of CML. Imatinib inhibits the *bcr-abl* tyrosine kinase by preventing ATP attachment. Without ATP as phosphate donor, phosphorylation by *bcr-abl* tyrosine kinase is interrupted.
- The Philadelphia chromosome is also seen in acute lymphoblastic leukaemia

Chronic Myeloid Leukaemia (CML)

- In the UK there are approximately 600 new cases of CML each year. Incidence is about 1-2 per 100,000.

- Three distinct phases are recognised in CML: chronic, accelerated and blast crisis.
- Chronic phase (3-5 years duration): this is the initial phase
- Accelerated phase (2-15 months duration): this is an intermediate phase which is seen in two thirds of patients; others pass straight to a blast crisis phase.
- Blast crisis phase (3-6 months duration): ending in patient death
- The treatment options include: hydroxycarbamide (hydroxyurea) or busulfan, α-interferon, bone marrow transplantation, and imatinib.
- Interferon is treatment of choice for those who are elderly or do not have a matched bone marrow donor and is given after inducing remission with hydroxycarbamide (hydroxyurea).
- Leucophoresis lowers white cell count and alleviates symptoms of hyperviscosity.
- Radiotherapy may reduce painful enlarged spleens.
- In the UK the National Institute on Clinical Excellence (NICE) has produced guidelines on the use of Imatinib: *www.nice.org.uk*. Imatinib is used in adults with Ph[1] positive CML in the following situations: 1) in the chronic phase if they are either intolerant or have failed to respond to α-interferon; 2) in the accelerated or blast crisis phase provided they have not received it at an earlier stage. Imatinib is given orally 400 mg od (chronic phase) or 600mg od (accelerated and blast crisis phase). The haematological response to imatinib (i.e. the normalisation of the blood count) is about 90% of patients in the chronic phase; 50% in the accelerated phase; and 30% in the blast crisis phase. Complete cytogenetic response (i.e. the disappearance of Ph[1] bearing white cells) is 40% of patients in the chronic phase; 20% in the accelerated phase; and 5% in the blast crisis phase.

Philadelphia Chromosome (Ph¹)

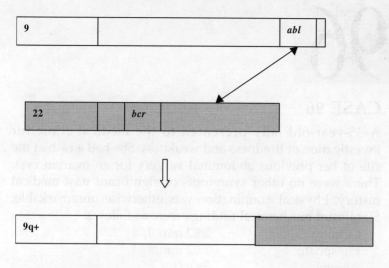

-333-

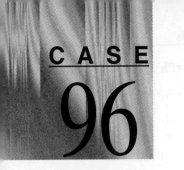

CASE 96

A 35-year-old lady presented to the medical clinic for investigation of tiredness and weakness. She had a rash at the site of her previous abdominal surgery for an ovarian cyst. There were no other symptoms or significant past medical history. Physical examination was otherwise unremarkable. Significant biochemical findings were as follows:

Calcium	2.82 mmol/l
Phosphate	1.02 mmol/l
Albumin	39 g/l

The medical registrar admitted the patient and commenced an oral medication. After 3 days the serum calcium was 2.24 mmol/l.

Questions
1. What was the diagnosis?
2. What was the oral medication?

Answers

1. Sarcoidosis
2. Prednisolone

The most common causes of hypercalcaemia are malignancy and hyperparathyroidism. Other causes include sarcoidosis, vitamin D intoxication and milk-alkali syndrome. However, this patient did not have symptoms suggestive of milk-alkali syndrome and she was not taking any medications. The normal serum phosphate makes hyperparathyroidism unlikely.

Hypercalcaemia in sarcoidosis often occurs after holidays or during the summer months. This is due to excess vitamin D precursor, which is formed in the skin following sunlight exposure, and its conversion to 1,25 (OH) vitamin D by granulomas. The PTH is suppressed. Serum calcium levels will decline with corticosteroid or bisphosphonate therapy. In this patient skin biopsy of the rash confirmed the diagnosis of sarcoidosis.

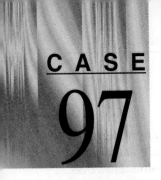

CASE 97

A 69-year-old man was referred to the hospital clinic with a history of hypertension. He was a non-smoker and did not consume alcohol. He had a hip replacement 6 months ago. There was no family history of cardiovascular illnesses. His blood pressure was noted to be elevated on many previous occasions by his General Practitioner. He subsequently started recording his own blood pressure at home, and the results were always less than 140/80 mmHg. The General Practitioner was, therefore, uncertain on the need for antihypertensive treatment. At the out patient clinic his blood pressure was 180/92 mmHg. There were no cardiac murmurs, the lungs were clear, and general examination was unremarkable. Chest X-ray, ECG, urinalysis, and routine blood test were all normal. The patient was fitted with an ambulatory blood pressure monitor (ABPM) at 11.30 hours in the hospital clinic. The results are displayed below.

Summary over 24 hours

	Min	Mean	Max	SD
Systolic (mmHg)	105	137	199	24.32
Diastolic (mmHg)	51	71	95	11.65
MAP (mmHg)	73	95	127	15.9
Heart Rate (bpm)	56	67	93	9.36

Percent of Systolic Readings above period limits: 28%
Percent of Diastolic Readings above period limits: 12%
Percent of time Systolic was above period limits: 24.8%
Percent of time Diastolic was above period limits: 10.2%
Key: SD = standard deviation
      bpm = beats per minute
      MAP = mean arterial pressure

Summary: 06:00 to 21:00 hours

	Min	Mean	Max	SD
Systolic (mmHg)	122	149	199	22.30
Diastolic (mmHg)	64	78	95	8.91
MAP (mmHg)	36	104	127	13.12
Heart Rate (bpm)	56	71	93	8.96

Percent of Systolic Readings > 140 mmHg:	43.8 %
Percent of Diastolic Readings > 85 mmHg:	18.8 %
Percent of time Systolic > 140 mmHg:	36.9 %
Percent of time Diastolic > 85 mmHg:	15.1 %

Summary: 21:00 to 06:00 hours

	Min	Mean	Max	SD
Systolic (mmHg)	105	117	128	8.47
Diastolic (mmHg)	51	60	67	5.21
MAP (mmHg)	73	80	90	6.35
Heart Rate (bpm)	56	60	72	5.15

Percent of Systolic Readings > 140 mmHg:	0.0 %
Percent of Diastolic Readings > 85 mmHg:	0.0 %
Percent of time Systolic > 140 mmHg:	0.0 %
Percent of time Diastolic > 85 mmHg:	0.0 %

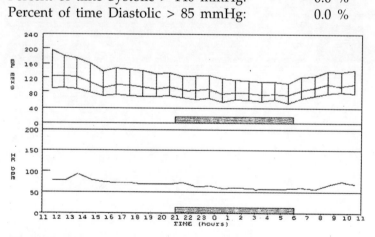

Questions

1. What does the ABPM recording show?
2. What is the diagnosis?

Answers

1. The ABPM shows a high clinic blood pressure reading that settles down gradually and dips at night time.
2. White coat hypertension

White Coat Hypertension

White coat hypertension is defined as a blood pressure ≥ 140/90 mmHg when measured in a clinic or office setting with a normal daytime ABPM readings < 135/85 mmHg. The prevalence is about 15-30% in the general population and is commonly seen in elderly people and pregnant women. The cardiovascular risks are considerably less compared to those with sustained hypertension and this should help to reassure individuals and insurers. However, patients need to be followed up due to the possibility that this could be a precursor to developing hypertension later. This condition has to be considered in newly diagnosed hypertensives and before prescribing drugs.

CASE 98

A 60-year-old lady presented with acute onset chest pain. The ECG is shown below.

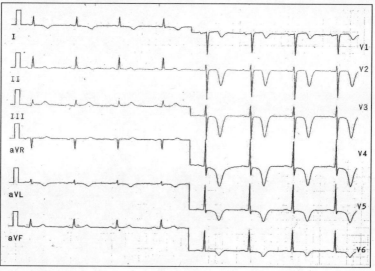

Questions

1. What does the ECG show?
2. What is the diagnosis?

Answers

1. The ECG shows:
   - Sinus bradycardia
   - Symmetrical 'T' inversion in lead I and aVL and V1 to V6

2. Acute non-Q wave myocardial infarction (non-STEMI). The term 'acute coronary syndrome' (ACS) refers to three clinical entities: unstable angina, non-Q myocardial infarction (or non-STEMI) and ST elevation myocardial infarction (or STEMI).

99

CASE 99

A 45-year-old man was admitted to hospital with a stroke. A week later he suddenly became breathless. He was tachycardic with an oxygen saturation of 85% and an ECG was performed and shown below (ECG 1).

ECG 1

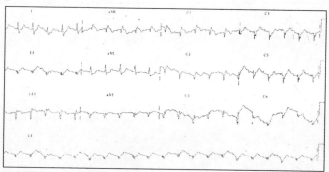

He was treated appropriately and a repeat ECG was obtained three days later (ECG 2).

ECG 2

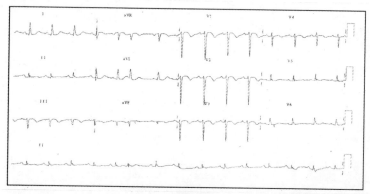

Questions

1. What does ECG 1 show?
2. What does ECG 2 show?
3. What is possible cause of his breathlessness?

Answers

1. ECG 1 shows:
   - Sinus tachycardia
   - 'S' in lead I, 'Q' and 'T' inversion in lead III (S1 Q3 T3 pattern)
   - 'Q' in anterior leads
   - ST elevation in VI
2. ECG 2 shows:
   - T flattening or inversion in inferior leads and anterior chest leads
3. Acute pulmonary embolism

ECG in pulmonary embolism shows:
a. Right atrial dilatation - tall T wave in lead II
b. Right ventricular strain - right bundle branch block, right axis deviation and T inversion in right precordial leads

The S1 Q3 T3 pattern is rare in pulmonary embolism.

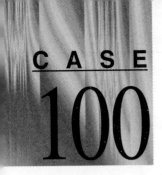

CASE 100

A 50-year-old man presented with acute onset chest pain. The ECG is shown below.

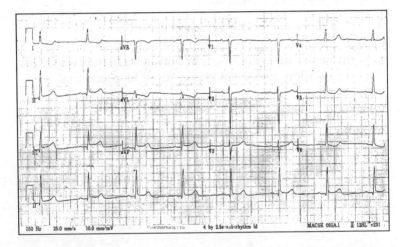

Questions
1. What does the ECG show?
2. What is the diagnosis?

Answers

1. The ECG shows:
   - Sinus bradycardia
   - ST elevation and Q waves in leads II, III and aVF
2. Acute inferior myocardial infarction

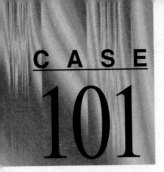

CASE 101

A 70-year-old man presented with acute onset chest pain. The ECG is shown below.

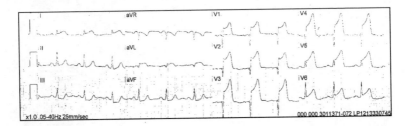

Questions
1. What does the ECG show?
2. What is the diagnosis?

Answers

1. The ECG shows:
   - ST elevation and Q waves in anterolateral chest leads
2. Acute anterolateral myocardial infarction

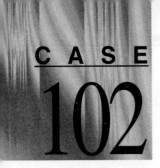

CASE 102

A 35-year-old lady presented with long standing breathlessness. Clinically she had a systolic murmur in the pulmonary area. Her 12 lead ECG is shown below.

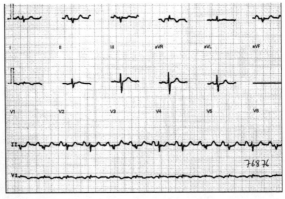

Question
What does the ECG show?

Answer

1. The ECG shows dominant 'P' wave in lead II suggestive of right atrial enlargement

Right atrial enlargement is seen in conditions like:

1. Primary pulmonary hypertension
2. Secondary pulmonary hypertension
   - Chronic lung disorders (bronchiectasis, COPD, pulmonary fibrosis)
   - Multiple pulmonary embolism
   - Kyphoscoliosis
3. Cardiac conditions
   - Atrial septal defect
   - Pulmonary stenosis

Each medical institution will have its own reference values. The following table is for guidance only.

Normal Values in SI units

Adrenocorticotrophic hormone	ACTH	10-80 ng/l
Alkaline phosphatase	ALP	35-130 U/l
Aminotransferase:	AST	10-40 U/l
(or transaminase)	ALT	5-40 U/l
Arterial blood gases (on air):	pH	7.35-7.45
	PaO_2	10-13 kPa
	$PaCO_2$	4.5-6.0 kPa
Bicarbonate	HCO_3	22-30 mmol/l
Bilirubin:	Total	3-17 µmol/l
	Conjugated	< 3.4 µmol/l
Calcium (corrected)	Ca	2.20-2.65 mmol/l
Chloride	Cl	95-105 mmol/l
Creatinine		60-120 µmol/l
Creatine kinase:	Men	30-220 U/l
	Women	20-170 U/l
Ferritin		20-300 µg/l
Folate:	Plasma	5-40 nmol/l
	Red cell	770-1800 nmol/l
γ-glutamyl transpeptidase	γ-GT	7-32 U/l
Magnesium	Mg	0.7-1.1 mmol/l
Plasma osmolality		280-296 mosmol/kg
Phosphate	PO_4	0.8-1.4 mmol/l
Potassium	K	3.5-5.0 mmol/l
Protein:	Albumin	35-50 g/l
	Globulin	20-25 g/l
Parathyroid hormone	PTH	1.6-6.9 pmol/l
Sodium	Na	135-145 mmol/l
Thyrotropin	TSH	0.4-5.0 mU/l
Total thyroxine	TT4	70-140 nmol/l
Free thyroxine	FT4	12.0-23.0 pmol/l
Total T3	TT3	1.2-3.0 nmol/l
Free T3	FT3	4.0-7.8 pmol/l
Urea		2.5-6.7 mmol/l
Total cholesterol		3.5-6.5 mmol/l (ideal < 5.0 mmol/l)
LDL cholesterol		1.5-4.4 mmol/l (ideal < 3.0 mmol/l)
HDL cholesterol:	Men	0.9-1.7 mmol/l (ideal > 1.0 mmol/l)
	Women	1.0-2.2 mmol/l (ideal > 1.0 mmol/l)
Triglycerides:	Men	0.7-2.2 mmol/l (ideal < 1.7 mmol/l)
	Women	0.6-1.7 mmol/l (ideal < 1.7 mmol/l)
Haemoglobin:	Men	14.0-17.7 g/dl
	Women	12.2-15.2 g/dl
WBC		4.0-10.0 x 10^9/l
Platelets		150-400 x 10^9/l
MCV		80-96 fl
MCHC		32-35 g/dl
ESR		< 20 mm/h
Prothrombin time		10.7-13 seconds
Activated Partial Thromboplastin Time		25-33 seconds
Fibrin Degradation Products		< 5 µg/ml
D-dimers		< 0.5 µg/ml
Vitamin B_{12}		130-660 pmol/l
25(OH) vitamin D		20-110 nmol/l

Urinary calcium   2.5-7.5 mmol/day
Urinary free cortisol   50-180 nmol/day
Urinary 5HIAA   < 50 µmol/day

Numerical Abbreviations

Abbreviation	Symbol	Value		Example	
deci	d	10^{-1}	1/10	dl	decilitre
centi	c	10^{-2}	1/100	cm	centimetre
milli	m	10^{-3}	1/1,000	mmol	millimole
micro	µ	10^{-6}	1/1,000,000	µmol	micromole
nano	n	10^{-9}	1/1,000,000,000	nmol	nanomole
pico	p	10^{-12}	1/1,000,000,000,000	pmol	picomole
femto	f	10^{-15}	1/1,000,000,000,000,000	fl	femtolitre

ILLUSTRATIONS

(* these illustrations are found in the answers section)

ACKNOWLEDGEMENTS

The authors are extremely grateful to colleagues in the Medical Photography Department at Basildon University Hospital for their help in producing these illustrations.

INTERNET RESOURCES

The following websites provide an extensive catalogue of medical reviews. Basic information is provided by the online version of the Merck manual. In depth articles from Emedicine and Medscape are constantly updated. Bandolier provides succinct summaries of the latest evidence based medicine. Registered users of Medscape and Mdlinx receive regular emails that contain information on the latest articles selected from a wide range of medical journals. Registration is not always required and at present access to these sites is free of charge.
www.emedicine.com
www.medscape.com
www.postgradmed.com
www.mdlinx.com
www.merck.com/pubs/mmanual
www.jr2.ox.ac.uk/bandolier

The following websites provide up to date information on health care guidelines that are used in the UK:
www.nice.org.uk
www.bnf.org.uk
www.hyp.ac.uk/bhs/resources/guidelines.htm
www.dvla.gov.uk
www.rcplondon.ac.uk

General purpose search engine:
www.google.com

General medicine journal:
www.bmj.com

HANDHELD COMPUTER SOFTWARE WEBSITES

The following websites provide free software for use in handheld computers, including medical calculators and patient tracking systems:
www.palmgear.com
www.memoware.com
www.handheldmed.com
http://5star.freeserve.com/PDA
www.handango.com